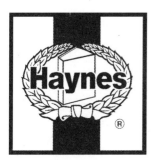

D0507802

The Cancer
Manual

Dr Ian Banks

Cartoons by Jim Campbell

Models Covered
Various, all shapes, sizes and colours

(4158 - 160)

ABCDE
FGHIJ
KLMNO
PQRST

Printed by **J H Haynes & Co Ltd,**
Sparkford, Yeovil, Somerset BA22 7JJ, England.

Haynes Publishing
Sparkford, Yeovil, Somerset BA22 7JJ, England

Haynes North America, Inc
861 Lawrence Drive, Newbury Park, California 91320, USA

Editions Haynes
4, Rue de l'Abreuvoir
92415 COURBEVOIE CEDEX, France

Haynes Publishing Nordiska AB
Box 1504, 751 45 UPPSALA, Sverige

ISBN **1 84425 158 6**

British Library Cataloguing in Publication Data
A catalogue record for this book is available from the British Library.

250 541 329

HAYNES PUBLISHING: MORE THAN JUST MANUALS

Haynes Publishing Group is the worldwide market leader in the production and sale of car and motorcycle repair manuals. Every vehicle manual is based on a complete strip-down and rebuild in our workshops. This approach, reflecting thoroughness and attention to detail, is integral to all our publications.

The Group publishes many other DIY titles as well as an extensive array of books about motor sport, vehicles and transport in general. Through its subsidiary Sutton Publishing the Group has also extended its interests to include history books.

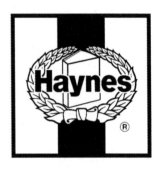

MHF

The Men's Health Forum is a charity that aims to improve men's health in England and Wales through:

Research and policy development
Professional training
Providing information services
Stimulating professional and public debate
Working with MPs and Government
Developing innovative and imaginative projects
Collaborating with the widest possible range of interested organisations and individuals
Organising the annual National Men's Health Week

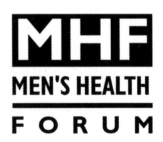

Contents

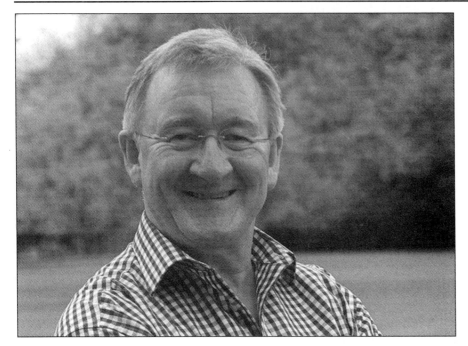

Men and cancer sounds so depressing, yet the big killers of men such as lung and bowel cancer are either preventable or easily treatable when caught early. In my work as a practising GP, many men unfortunately come to see me later rather than sooner. I use television to encourage men to use their doctor as a source of good advice and early diagnosis. Men's health matters, particularly when it comes to prevention and early diagnosis of cancer. Use this manual just as you would use any other source of good information and act on what it recommends. When it comes to cancer, us owners of the Y chromosome should be the first to ask why.

Dr Chris Steele

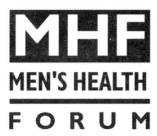

The author, the publisher and the Men's Health Forum would like to thank the following organisations for their contributions to the content, production and distribution of this manual.

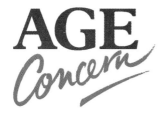

Age Concern

Age Concern campaigns and works for everybody's future. The issues affecting older people today concern us all. We work all over the country making more of life for older people and are supported by a vibrant network of volunteers.

Nationally, we take a lead role in campaigning, parliamentary work, policy analysis, research, specialist information and advice provision, and a wide range of training.

Innovative programmes provide healthier lifestyles and provide older people with opportunities to give the experience of a lifetime back to their communities.

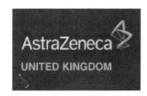

AstraZeneca

AstraZeneca provides new and effective prescription medicines that make a real difference for patients. We concentrate on important areas of medical need: cancer, cardiovascular disease and mental health.

We employ 10,000 people in the UK in eight principal sites including two research and development centres at Alderley Park in Cheshire and Charnwood in Leicestershire.

Innovation and creativity are strong themes in our business. Thanks to the ideas and energy of our people, we have one of the best new product pipelines in the industry, enabling us to make a real difference.

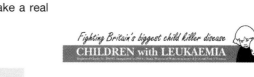

Beating Bowel Cancer

Beating Bowel Cancer is a national charity working to raise awareness of symptoms, promote early diagnosis and encourage open access to treatment choice for those affected by bowel cancer – the second biggest cause of cancer deaths in the UK.

The charity was founded in 1999 and is based in Middlesex. It aims to improve bowel cancer awareness amongst both the medical profession and the general public - providing authoritative information about the disease. The charity encourages people to communicate frankly and not to be embarrassed to talk about bottoms and bowels!

It relies almost entirely upon donations and a network of fundraisers across the country.

Children With Leukaemia

CWL was established in 1988 in memory of Paul O'Gorman who lost his fight against leukaemia at only 14 years of age and his sister Jean who died of breast cancer only nine months later.

What started as a small memorial charity is now Britain's leading charity dedicated exclusively to the conquest of childhood leukaemia through pioneering research into the causes of and treatments for leukaemia and the support of leukaemic children and their families.

GUS plc

GUS plc is a retail and business services group which provides information and customer relationship management services through Experian, general merchandise through ARG (which includes Argos and Homebase)and luxury goods through a majority shareholding in Burberry Group plc. GUS employs over 32,500 men.

A wide range of charitable projects are supported with information and resources, most of which are channelled through the GUS Charitable Trust. The Trust initiated and currently supports the work of the Prostate Cancer Charter for Action, a campaigning partnership of charities and professional groups with an interest in prostate cancer.

The Prostate Cancer Charter for Action is backed by all the key professional and charity organisations with an interest in prostate cancer, who have joined together to speak with one voice. Imitated and launched with generous support from the GUS Charitable Trust, the Charter calls for action on transparency, public awareness, patient care, resources and partnership.

The GUS Charitable Trust's commitment to men's health includes substantial backing for this book.

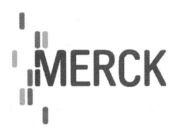

MERCK Oncology

Founded in 1668 in Darmstadt, Germany, Merck is a leading pharmaceutical and chemical company operating in 55 countries with more than 34,000 employees.

Merck Pharmaceuticals is committed to addressing unmet medical needs in crucial areas, such as cancer.

Our oncology projects focus on novel biotherapeutic strategies that represent more selective modes of tumour destruction and have few side-effects.

Through our own research capabilities and strategic alliances, eight potential cancer drugs have been advanced to various stages of clinical development. Our Oncology portfolio is based on four innovative approaches:
- Monoclonal antibodies.
- Cancer vaccines.
- Angiogenesis inhibitors.
- Immunocytokines.

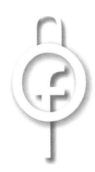

The National Obesity Forum (NOF)

NOF is an independent medical organisation, whose aim is to raise the awareness of obesity as a serious medical condition and to promote best quality management within the NHS. The NOF provides evidence based clinical guidelines for medical management of adult obesity, childhood obesity (in association with the Royal College of Paediatrics and Child Health) and for pharmacotherapy for obesity, which have been widely published and utilised by health authorities within the UK and internationally. We award the annual "Award for Excellence in Obesity Management in Primary Care" and have published educational material for all healthcare professionals on paper, CDRom and on our website. There is an annual NOF conference on the clinical management of obesity. The NOF is a first port of call for professional advice to the media on all obesity related issues. The NOF helped establish the All Party Parliamentary Group on Obesity in 2002, continues to provide professional and secretarial support to the Chairs, Dr Howard Stoate MP and Mr Vernon Coaker MP, facilitating four parliamentary meetings each year, and we have provided expert opinion for the National Institute for Clinical Excellence (NICE).

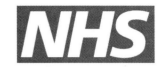

The NHS

The National Health Service was set up in 1948 to provide healthcare for all citizens, based on need, not the ability to pay. It is made up of a wide range of health professionals, support workers and organisations.

The NHS aims to bring about the highest level of physical and mental health for all citizens, within the resources available, by:
- Promoting health and preventing ill-health.
- Diagnosing and treating injury and disease.
- Caring for those with a long-term illness and disability, who require the services of the NHS.

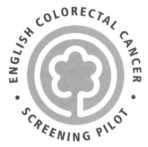

The NHS Cancer Screening Programmes

The NHS Cancer Screening Programmes comprises two nationally co-ordinated screening programmes for breast and cervical cancer, the English Bowel Screening Pilot and Prostate Cancer Risk Management. The programme operates on the principle of *Informed Choice*, providing men and women with clear and balanced information from which they can make informed decisions about their health. Prostate Cancer Risk Management provides resources to enable men considering a prostate specific antigen (PSA) test to be given information concerning the benefits, limitation and risks associated with receiving a test, while the English Bowel Screening Pilot is evaluating the practicalities involved in implementing a national screening programme.

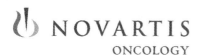

NOVARTIS

Novartis AG (NYSE: NVS) is a world leader in pharmaceuticals and consumer health. In 2002, the Group's businesses achieved sales of CHF 32.4 billion (USD 20.9 billion) and a net income of CHF 7.3 billion (USD 4.7 billion). The Group invested approximately CHF 4.3 billion (USD 2.8 billion) in R&D. Headquartered in Basel, Switzerland, Novartis Group companies employ about 72 900 people and operate in over 140 countries around the world.

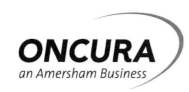

ONCURA

ONCURA, a Global Leader in Minimally Invasive Prostate Cancer Disease Management.

ONCURA is a newly formed company resulting from the merger of Amersham's brachytherapy business with Galil Medical Ltd's cryotherapy business. ONCURA combines the market leadership of Amersham in brachytherapy with the rapidly growing area of cryotherapy.

ONCURA provides exclusive 3rd Generation Cryotherapy technology through the SeedNet™Gold Cryotherapy system and unique ultra-thin 17 gauge CryoNeedles™ as well as leading prostate brachytherapy seed products – RAPID Strand™, OncoSeed™, EchoSeed™ and TheraSeed®. In addition ONCURA will also offer the option of cryotherapy for the treatment of kidney cancer.

The Orchid Cancer Appeal

Formed in 1996 the Orchid Cancer Appeal was the first registered charity dedicated to funding research into diagnosis, prevention and treatment of both testicular and prostate cancer as well as promoting awareness of these previously neglected diseases.

As well as funding cutting edge

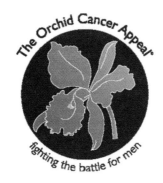

research into men's cancers the Orchid Cancer Appeal has produced a range of leaflets and other resource material free of charge to help people understand these cancers and their treatment.

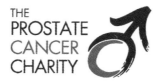

The Prostate Cancer Charity

The Prostate Cancer Charity provides support and information for men with prostate cancer, their families and the public, raises awareness of the condition, and funds scientific research into all aspects of the disease, including screening, diagnosis and treatment. The Charity produces a wide range of literature, free on request, runs a confidential telephone Helpline service staffed by nurses and has an extensive website. It also has a nationwide network of support contacts and volunteers.

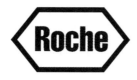

Roche

Roche aims to improve the health, quality of life and wellbeing of people in the UK through its innovative range of diagnostic, pharmaceutical and consumer health products that focus on the needs of individuals.

This breadth of interest enables us to take an integrated approach to healthcare, focusing on the prevention, diagnosis and treatment of disease and the enhancement of well-being.

Part of one of the world's leading healthcare companies, Roche is proud to have been a part of the UK's healthcare environment since 1908. Today we employ around 1,800 people based at two main sites in Welwyn Garden City, Hertfordshire, and Lewes, East Sussex.

Royal Mail Group plc

Royal Mail Group plc operates as three well-known and trusted businesses: Royal Mail, Post Office®, and Parcelforce Worldwide, with a turnover of £8 billion.

Royal Mail's 140,000 postmen and women use a fleet of 30,000 vehicles, 33,000 bicycles - and their feet - to collect, sort and deliver 82 million letters each day to the nation's 27 million addresses.

Parcelforce Worldwide's employees operate in the fiercely competitive market for express deliveries, and Post Office® employees run the UK's largest retail chain providing 170 products and services to 28 million customers each week.

As the largest employers of men in the UK, their health is vital to our success, and we are delighted to support this manual.

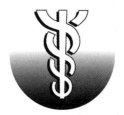

World Cancer Research Fund

World Cancer Research Fund (WCRF UK) is the only major UK registered charity dedicated solely to the prevention of cancer through healthy diets and lifestyles. WCRF UK is committed to providing cancer research and education programmes which expand our understanding of the importance of food and lifestyle choices in the cancer process. By spreading the good news that cancer can be prevented, WCRF UK believes that many thousands of lives will be saved. The work of WCRF UK is funded solely by donations from the public.

Author's acknowledgements

The author would like to thank all those who have helped in putting this manual together. Jim Campbell's cartoons have done much to lighten what can be somewhat gloomy topics. Ian Barnes and Matthew Minter have brought Haynes standards to bear on the raw material; Dr. Simon Gregory was referred to for a second opinion.

As for the raw material itself, I must extend my grateful thanks to the following specialist contributors, and my apologies to anyone who has been accidentally omitted from the list:

- Alan White for European statistics on men and cancer
- Caroline Beswick, Trinity PR (on behalf of Beating Bowel Cancer) for the bowel cancer material.
- Chris Hiley (Head of Policy and Research, The Prostate Cancer Charity) for the material on prostate cancer.
- Colin Osborne (President and Founder, The Orchid Cancer Appeal) for the material on testicular cancer.
- David Haslam and Ian Campbell for the material on obesity.
- David Haslam for the material on cancer quackery.
- Professor Denis Henshaw, of the University of Bristol, for the material on electromagnetic radiation.
- Jim Pollard of the Men's Health Forum for the Cancer on the Web section.
- Maebh Jennins for WCRF UK's section on cancer prevention.
- Matthew Maycock of the Men's Health Forum for contacts & addresses.
- Sara Hawksworth and Carolyn Robertson, both from the ActivAge Unit at Age Concern England, for the material on cancer and older men.
- Dr Steven Boorman MBBS MRCGP FFOM, specialist occupational physician and Chief Medical Adviser to the Royal Mail Group, for the material on Cancer and Occupation.
- Mr Tim Lane FRCS, consultant urologist, for the material on kidney, bladder and penile cancer

Man and His Machine

Man #1 has been around for a very long time. As the proud owner of the latest model you'll be keen to keep it in top condition. With a little care your high performance machine will last you a long lifetime with minimal need for maintenance or spare parts. But like any sophisticated piece of high technology, your body will respond best to a basic understanding of what goes on underneath the bonnet.

In truth, men are more likely to look after their cars than their own bodies. Of course, MOTs are required by law for your car but there is no such equivalent for the driver. However, many illnesses can be prevented and with early diagnosis, successfully treated. Cancer is a prime example of this. This manual arms you with the information you need to keep your body humming like a finely tuned engine, so you can reduce your risk, and where possible, prevent cancer. It also gives you the tools to notice early warning signs that need to be checked out, so that little problems don't become big problems. Should the big ends need attention it looks at what can be done and the impact this can have on fellow passengers. This is not a doom and gloom manual. It is optimistic for all the right reasons. Men do not have to die early especially from cancer.

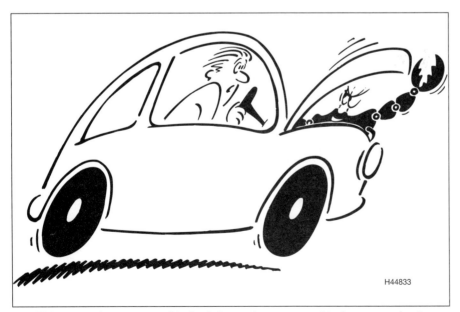

H44833

This manual arms you with the information you need to keep your body humming like a finely tuned engine

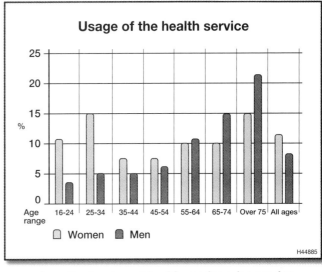

Usage of the health service

Consultation with a GP, by gender

Usage of the health service

In-patient usage of health services, by gender

It's not just men in the UK either, across the whole of Europe men go far too late when they find something wrong. There is an average delay of 14 weeks between a young man finding a lump on his testicle and going to see his doctor. Worse still, the deadly skin cancer melanoma is very unforgiving when it comes to late presentation to a doctor. Despite the fact that more women across Europe develop melanoma, more men die from it.

This is true for every cancer common to both sexes. Although in many cases men also develop cancer more often than do women, this simply makes going to see your doctor late even more dangerous.

As a result not only do men tend to die earlier than do women they also end up in hospital more often in their later life.

So the message is loud and clear, when you find something wrong go and get it checked out. There is a great deal you can do for yourself, not least in preventing cancer in the first place. All the major charities and organisations involved with cancer and men contributed to the various sections. You will not get a better insight into what you can do about cancer. By following the guidelines in this manual you can be more than just a bog standard model. You can be more, much more. You can be a highly tuned man machine. And you might just reach retirement age as a highly prized vintage model in A1 order.

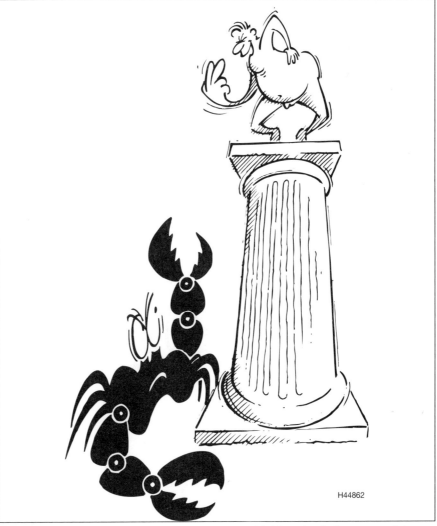

You might just reach retirement age as a highly prized vintage model in A1 order

0•10 **Notes**

Chapter 1
Men and cancer

Contents

1 Introduction

Cancer is common and because we are generally living longer it's becoming commoner. Although no one would deny that most cancers are serious, the idea that a diagnosis of cancer is a certain death warrant is now far from the truth. Most cancer deaths are avoidable through prevention or early diagnosis.

Cancer covers about 200 different diseases, and although about one man in three will develop a cancer at some time in his life, the most common forms are almost entirely preventable or treatable through early diagnosis.

With the exception of cancer of the breast, thyroid and skin (melanoma), all cancers are commoner in men than in women. Cancer of the bladder is nearly four times as common in men; lung cancer is three and a half times as common; stomach cancer is two and a half times as common; mouth, gullet and kidney cancers are twice as common; and colorectal, pancreas, brain, lymph and various other cancers are one and a half times as common. Being a man could seriously damage your health unless we recognise the risks.

Misunderstanding is the real curse of cancer, with loads of problems over terminology. For instance, the difference between tumours and cancers is important. In general terms a tumour is any sort of body swelling but the word is now commonly used in conjunction with cancer. Basically, all cancers are tumours, but not all tumours are cancers. This is important as many men will pick up the wrong message when talking to their doctors.

There are two types of tumours and they can be very different when it comes to potential harm and treatment.

Benign tumours

Benign tumours are not cancers. They are clumps of cells arising from tissues such as muscle, nerve, fat, blood vessels which have begun to reproduce and multiply more rapidly than normal. The most important point is that they don't spread to other parts of the body. Even so, the term 'benign tumour' can be misleading. They are only benign in the sense that they stay in the same place and don't spread to other parts of the body. Not that this means they are harmless. Sometimes they grow very large and can put pressure on vital organs, particularly when within the skull. Many brain tumours are benign, but because of their situation and the fact that there is no room for them to expand, they can do a lot of harm. The good news is that they never spread their way into other tissues and they never bud off elsewhere.

Malignant tumours

Malignant tumours are the 'true' cancers and they behave quite differently from benign tumours. Although there are a large number of types they can be grouped into two broad classes.

Surface linings

These are the commonest and are called carcinomas (carcin- means 'hard' and -oma means 'a lump').

Any lining surface, anywhere in the body, can become the site of a carcinoma. So in men they can arise, for instance, in the skin, the stomach, the colon (large bowel), the rectum (lower end of large bowel), the prostate gland, the bronchial tubes, the ducts of the pancreas or gall bladder, or the breast.

Solid tissues

These are called sarcomas (sarc- means 'flesh') and they are much less common than carcinomas, except in people with AIDS. They arise in muscle, bone, lymph nodes, blood vessels, and fibrous and other connective tissues.

Both carcinomas and sarcomas have the dangerous property of invasiveness. Instead of forming isolated lumps in a capsule like benign tumours, they burrow into and invade adjacent tissues and structures, often destroying them.

As a cancer grows it can burrow through the wall of a blood vessel and then be carried off by the fast-flowing blood to remote parts of the body. This process is called metastasis. The new lump of growing cancer caused in this way is also called a metastasis. Some cancers seem to have preferred places to grow once travelling around the body. This is the main reason why cancers are so serious. They are always liable, by metastasis, to send off cancer cells to other places in the body. Thus a cancer

1

in the lung or colon or prostate can be transported to the brain or bones or liver, to set up a new focus and continue to grow and invade in the new site.

Just to make things even worse, there are thin-walled tubes throughout the body, called lymphatic ducts. These carry off excess fluid from the tissues back to the bloodstream. Lymphatics are very easily invaded by cancers, and this is a very common way for cancer cells to spread. Cancers spreading to lymphatic ducts are held up, for a time, in the lymph nodes. Treatment of spreading cancer can depend on the spread to these nodes.

Speed

Not all cancers are the same in their ability to spread quickly, or in the readiness with which they form new colonies elsewhere. This tendency is called malignancy and malignancy may be low or high. A tumour of low malignancy may take many months or even years to cause any trouble and may not spread distantly for a very long time, if ever. This is seen very often with prostate cancer. Unfortunately, tumours of high malignancy will sometimes spread widely before the man sees his doctor.

Body defences

Cancer cells are often recognized as 'foreign' by a healthy immune system and attacked. People whose immune systems have been damaged, whether by AIDS or any other cause, are much more liable than normal to acquire cancer. Most of us probably develop and overcome cancer many times in our lifetime without ever realising it.

Even so, the immune system can't do much about a cancer that has grown beyond a critical size and this is where early diagnosis is so important.

Causes

Once it was thought that there was one unifying cause for cancer and that finding this would solve the problem for all cancers. We now know that there are many causes, of which a large number remain uncertain. Cancer of the skin, for instance, can be caused by excessive exposure to sunlight but also by contact with certain toxic chemicals. Cancer of

the neck of the womb (cervix) is obviously not a male disease, yet it may be caused by a sexually transmitted virus which causes penile warts in men.

Similarly, not all cancers arise in the place where they cause the most trouble. Liver cancer, for instance, is relatively common but the cancer more usually comes by spreading from elsewhere such as the bowel. So far as the liver itself is concerned, conditions like cirrhosis or hepatitis B virus infection may lead to primary liver cancer. There is also a very strong link between liver cancer and a poison, aflatoxin, produced by a mould that grows on peanuts and grains in moist, warm areas.

Some causes were identified very early on and were linked to industrial

processes. Various forms of radiation cause cancer. Before this was understood, scores of women employed to paint the dials of watches and clocks with radium- or mesothorium-containing luminous paint died from cancers of the tongue and jaw. These women used to point their fine paint brushes by using their lips.

Many substances are known to cause skin cancer and these include soot, tar, creosote, pitch and various mineral oils. One of the greatest crimes of the so-called great Victorian era was to use young children to clean chimneys. They were often sent up while the chimney was still hot and suffered dreadful burns to their knees and hands which were scrubbed with salt to make

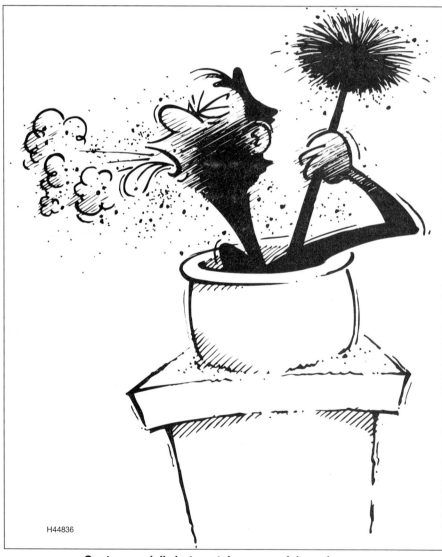

H44836

Soot, especially hot soot, is a powerful carcinogen

them 'tougher'. Soot, especially hot soot, is a powerful carcinogen and these poor boys often developed scrotal cancer, not to mention chest diseases which progressed to cancer. When shale oil was used to lubricate the high-speed spindles in the early cotton mills, a fine spray of oil used to soak the trousers of the mill workers and large numbers of them developed skin cancer of the scrotum in a similar way to child chimney sweeps.

A more modern cancer was denied for many years. Mesothelioma is an invariably fatal cancer of the lining of the lungs. Asbestos exposure is almost the only cause. As with asbestosis the link was well-recognised by men working in the industry, and the doctors treating them, but denied by the asbestos industry for legal and financial reasons. Now working with asbestos without adequate protection would be considered an act of great folly. Yet only a couple of decades ago workers in ship yards who fitted asbestos sheets to the ship's hulls and boiler rooms were called 'the White Men' because of the inevitable head-to-toe covering of asbestos with little or no protection. Tragically, wives of these men washing their overalls were also at risk and many died as a result.

Even the most innocuous industrial process can possess hidden dangers of cancer. Woodworkers were noticed to have a much higher incidence of nasal cancer than the general population, in which it is quite rare. Fine particles of wood dust are to blame and it took a while before the penny dropped. Unfortunately even when the cause of an industrial cancer is recognised the forms of protection can make things no better or even worse. A good example is overhead extractors, which bring the dangerous substances past the person's body before being removed from the area. Downward extractors keep the dust at ground level, reducing risk.

Sometimes there is a mixture of links which add up to increasing the risks of cancer quite considerably. Men who smoke, for instance, are at greater risk from some industrial carcinogenic chemicals. Not all chemicals are purely industrial, there can be overlaps, but the list of chemicals known to cause cancer is long and getting longer:

- Alcohol (cancers of mouth, throat, gullet and liver).
- Anabolic steroids (cancer of liver).
- Arsenic (cancers of lung, skin and liver).
- Chromium (cancer of lung).
- Isopropyl alcohol (cancer of nasal sinuses).
- Nickel dust (cancer of lung and sinuses).
- Phenacetin (cancer of kidney and bladder).
- Snuff-taking and tobacco chewing (cancer of mouth).
- Vinyl chloride (cancer of liver).

If history has taught us anything it is to treat all industrial processes with extreme caution, making best use of protective clothing, and reporting any health concerns to the management, occupational health service and trade union.

Tobacco smoking

Despite the bleating from the tobacco industry and their funded 'independent' advocacy groups, the evidence linking cancer of the lung to cigarette smoking is overwhelming. Most people, including governments, now accept this, but what many people don't realise is that smoking can also cause cancer of the tongue and bladder and in various other organs. The cancer-producing substances in cigarette smoke are absorbed into the blood and get everywhere in the body.

Normal cell DNA contains genes called proto-oncogenes. These remain harmless unless acted on by a carcinogen. When this happens, cancer-producing genes (oncogenes) are formed. Mutations in proto-oncogenes can also lead to cancer. One of the arguments is that tobacco doesn't actually cause cancer itself but instead triggers viruses or the oncogenes which then cause all the trouble. Actually it doesn't make much difference. Trying to decide whether it's your finger which

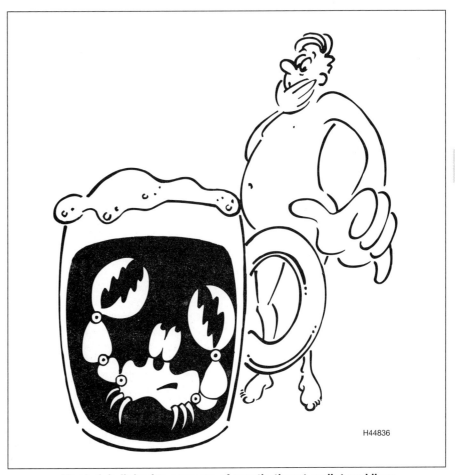

Alcohol is linked to cancers of mouth, throat, gullet and liver

H44836

1

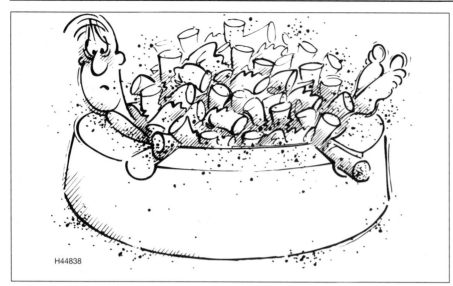

The cancer-producing substances in cigarette smoke are absorbed into the blood and get everywhere in the body

pulls the trigger of the gun or the bullet the gun fires that kills you is pretty academic. You still blow your head off.

Viruses

We do know that some viruses are associated with cancer. These are well-known viruses, such as the human papilloma (wart) virus, herpes viruses, the hepatitis B virus and HIV. Collectively, these are known as oncoviruses. One particular group of viruses, the retroviruses, contain genes that can, under certain circumstances, insert themselves into the genetic material (DNA) of normal cells triggering a cancerous growth pattern. Called 'oncogenes', even normal cells may also contain them and be triggered by these viruses.

Gene mutations

What is increasingly clear is the role of chemicals (carcinogens) that cause cancer through gene mutations. If this happens in cells such as the liver or bowel it can result in a tumour, but if it happens in one of the sex cells such as in the testes the mutation may be passed on to the next generation. This may be part of the reason why some cancers run in families. Strangely, although cancer cells appear very often in the body they may not actually go on to produce a full-blown tumour. It appears that other genes control these potentially dangerous genes suppressing their activity. These 'tumour suppressor genes' are vital and when they are damaged by chemicals or radiation it can lead to cancer. This may be the route that produces a cancer following treatment for other cancers such as the leukaemias (see Chapter 4). By a different route the body's own immune system can often recognise these tumour cells and destroy them before they grow to any size. A great deal of research is focused on exactly this aspect of our body's defence mechanism and why it can fail to recognise a tumour cell in the first place.

Early diagnosis

Obviously it is impossible to give one single way of diagnosing cancer as there are so many different kinds of cancer affecting different parts of the body. Early diagnosis is often the key to successful treatment and many cancers can be diagnosed by one or more of the following:

* Your symptoms, along with a doctor's clinical examination.
* Coughing or vomiting blood.
* Unexplained weight loss.
* Blood tests, especially microscopic examination.
* X-ray, CT or MRI scanning.
* Looking for the tumours using internal telescopes (endoscopes).
* Surgical exploratory operations. These are often combined with treatment.
* Laboratory tests for chemical substances called tumour markers.

Prevention

You might be surprised to know that some of the big cancers killers of men are either totally or partly preventable. See Chapter 2 for more information.

Treatment

As with diagnosis, cancer treatment varies with the different types. Look at the different Chapters for specific treatments. Although new forms of treatment come on stream all the time there are basically three principal forms of anticancer treatment:

* Surgery.
* Radiotherapy.
* Chemotherapy.

Surgery

Notwithstanding the huge advances in cancer treatment, the mainstay of cancer treatment is often surgery. Early surgery is just as important as for any form of treatment and if this can be done before a cancer has spread from its site of origin, the cancer is 'cured'. Once again the importance of turning up at your doctor's surgery early rather than late can make all the difference.

Surgery is no longer confined to those cases in which no evidence of remote spread (metastasis) could be found. Huge leaps forward in chemotherapy and other modes of cancer treatment mean it is now common to operate in selected cases to remove secondary liver tumours after removal of the primary cancer elsewhere in the body such as the bowel.

Radiotherapy

Here lies the true irony; radiation can cause cancer yet it can also cure it. Radiotherapy knocks out the atoms linking chemical molecules and so breaks them up. Although radiation affects both normal and cancerous tissues, almost all cancers are more sensitive to radiation and this is the key to destroying cancerous cells while sparing the normal cells. This subtle balancing act is dependent on the greater sensitivity of rapidly-dividing cells to radiation and the fact that, generally, cancer cells divide far more often than normal cells.

Long molecules like DNA are more susceptible to damage and this can disrupt the cancer cells' ability to survive. By shielding and focusing the radiation it can be directed accurately at a tumour with minimal exposure of non-malignant tissues so that a total dose of radiation can be applied to one localised area in levels which might otherwise be fatal. Getting the timing, intensity and direction of the doses of radiation is crucial for effective treatment and many of the great advances have taken place in this highly technological area.

Types of radiotherapy

Treatment will depend on the type and location of the tumour. Radiation sources used are high energy (high voltage) X-ray machines, linear accelerators and radioactive isotopes, such as cobalt-60 and iodine-131, which emit gamma rays. Lead shielding is used so that only the area of the tumour is irradiated and the dosage is usually spread over a period of some weeks. After each dose the effect is monitored to make sure that the right amount has been used. Checking on the way the bone marrow is behaving in producing vital blood cells for instance is one way of making sure too much radiation is not being used. A simple blood test will confirm optimum treatment.

Small and well-localised tumours can be effectively treated by direct application of radioactive sources in or around them. This is particularly useful for prostate cancer (see Chapter 7).

Around half of men needing radiotherapy will be cured, this is improved by early diagnosis which means getting to the doctor sooner rather than later. Radiotherapy can also make remaining life bearable even without a cure.

Chemotherapy

Huge advances are taking place in chemotherapy. Most anti-cancer drugs are cytotoxic drugs that destroy rapidly-growing cells, but a new class of drugs such as sex hormones or similar substances are increasingly being used to great effect.

Cytotoxic drugs are especially useful in the treatment of some forms of leukaemia, lymphomas, and testicular cancer. One of their great uses is as an additional safeguard after surgery or in conjunction with radiotherapy. Cytotoxic drugs cause more damage to cancer cells than normal body cells. As with radiotherapy most of the effect comes from distinguishing cancer cells from other cells by the speed with which cancer cells reproduce. Unfortunately this is not as precise as we would wish and they can have significant side effects, especially on those tissues which normally do divide rapidly anyway, including the blood-forming tissue in the bone marrow, the lining of the bowel, the hair-producing cells, and the sex glands. As a result chemotherapy can sometimes result in:

- Anaemia with easier bleeding than normal.
- A feeling of sickness (nausea) and vomiting.
- Hair loss (although this is by no means certain and can be very variable).
- Reduced fertility. Taking a sperm sample before treatment can ensure the chances of having children afterwards.

Frequent checks are therefore made of red and white blood cell counts during chemotherapy.

Some cancers like those of the prostate are 'hormone dependent' and certain hormones can make them grow faster. Inhibiting the production or action of testosterone can significantly reduce the rate at which the tumour grows (see Chapter 7).

2 Mister Myths

Remember the old 'myth' that cars can run on water and then they found out engines actually do work better in the rain because damp air makes the fuel burn more efficiently?

Well, cancer has its own myths and old wives' tales, some of which turn out to be partly true:

MYTH: Holding on too long before going for a pee causes bladder cancer.
- *No, but it can make you walk like John Wayne.*

MYTH: Artificial sweeteners cause bladder and bowel cancer.
- *This was a popular myth some time ago but is groundless.*

MYTH: Pesticides cause cancer.
- *A long runner this one but without good support. What we do know is there are undoubted links between many industrial chemicals and some cancers so if you work with these chemicals protective gear makes sense.*

MYTH: Masturbation causes testicular or prostate cancer.
- *Thankfully false. In fact there is evidence for the opposite and also for preventing impotence (erectile dysfunction). Use it or lose it.*

MYTH: Tight underpants cause testicular cancer.
- *False and yet falsetto.*

MYTH: Regularly eating meat cooked on a BBQ won't increase your risk for cancer.
- *False. Burnt meat is a real risk.*

MYTH: Men don't get breast cancer.
- *Sadly untrue but thankfully rare.*

MYTH: Women have prostates but they don't cause as much trouble.
- *Despite over 50% of men surveyed believing this to be true, it is false. Which is great news, otherwise two people would have to get up in the middle of the night.*

TRUTH: Tomatoes prevent prostate cancer.
- *Apparently true, with strong evidence for selenium and vitamin E as well.*

MYTH: If I have been diagnosed with prostate cancer, my wife will get cancer if I have sex with her.
- *False – you can't 'catch' cancer from someone else.*

MYTH: My prostate cancer will get worse if I have sex.
- *False – having sex has no effect on the progression of the cancer.*

MYTH: I feel well so I can't have cancer.
- *Not necessarily true – many cancers have no effect on the general health of the sufferer in their early stages.*

MYTH: I haven't lost any weight so I can't have cancer.
- *Not necessarily true – weight loss is not a feature of every type of cancer.*

MYTH: Electric and magnetic fields cause cancer.
- *The jury is out on this one. The following article is by Professor Denis Henshaw of the University of Bristol.*

1

Electricity and cancer

Electricity, where would we be without it? At the flick of a switch we produce light, activate a host of labour-saving devices and gadgets for our entertainment. While we use electricity in our 60 watt light bulbs, power companies routinely pump billions of watts around the country using high voltage powerlines. There is no question is there, electricity is clean and slick. After all, what possible dangers could there be in living with electricity?

We are now surrounded by vibrating electric and magnetic fields (EMFs) millions of times higher than those experienced by our predecessors just 100 years ago. It was only from the mid-1920s that mains electricity became widespread, and commercial radio started. Only 80 years ago there were virtually no man-made EMFs. Much of the United Kingdom still did not have an electricity supply, and in those areas which did, some were 'direct current' and did not vibrate many times every second. For example, much of rural Cambridgeshire did not receive an electricity supply until as recently as 1939.

By December 1932 the 'Wireless Constructor' was warning readers about the rise of radio transmissions: *"you may find yourself in the position of a paralysed man watching the rising of a tide which will ultimately drown him"*. Prophetic words?

Scientific research has associated male brain tumours, testicular tumours, breast cancer, leukaemias and ALS (a form of motor neurone disease) with electricity and microwaves. Is *"associated with"* the same as *"caused by"*?

It's almost impossible to find out whether long-term health effects are *caused* by *specific* environmental pollutants when "most people" are exposed "most of the time". Epidemiology (the study of illnesses in the general population) is good at identifying isolated and acute disease conditions. However the results are often misleading and inaccurate when applied to widespread, low-level, chronic conditions such as EMF exposure.

Human beings are complex and their response varies from individual to individual and within one individual over

their lifetime. Anticipating how one person will respond to a given stimulus is like trying to base a long-range weather forecast for the UK upon one drop of rain in East Anglia. The weather is an example of a complex system. Despite using expensive equipment, weather forecasters can still get it wrong, sometimes very wrong. Here we are trying to predict future health outcomes many years into the future. Many serious cancers are started up to 25 years before they are detected.

In fact there is now significant evidence that exposure to the electric and magnetic fields associated with power cables increases the risk of some types of cancer. The worries started with childhood leukaemia, but now scientists have found evidence of increased risk of some cancers in adults. All cables carrying electricity produce invisible electric and magnetic fields around them.

It is unlikely that EMFs cause cancer on their own. Most cancers are believed to start after a series of adverse things happen to living cells. Nuclear radiation (including X-rays) and some chemicals including tobacco smoke are known single causes. However, viruses, low levels of chemicals such as pesticides in food and EMFs have all been shown to play a possible role in the development of cancer. What is significant overall about the international studies is the suggestion that EMFs might increased the risk of some adult cancers.

Scientists have been unable to agree how EMFs may be involved in causing cancer. One particular mechanism which may be at work is via the disruption of the hormone melatonin in the body. In humans the main source of melatonin is its night-time production in the pineal gland, the production being triggered by a signal from the eye indicating the absence of light. A series of studies in humans has shown that magnetic fields as low as 0.2 µT also suppress nocturnal melatonin production. Melatonin is a particularly important hormone because of its property as a powerful natural anti-cancer agent. In the laboratory it has been shown to be highly protective of cancerous damage to cells in the blood and to impede the growth of breast cancer cells.

Scientists at Bristol University have been looking at ways in which electric fields associated with high voltage

powerlines may lead to a cancer risk. The high voltage carried by overhead powerline cables creates an intense electric field on their surfaces which can ionise the air, splitting it up into electrons, and nitrogen and oxygen ions. These ions are blown away from the powerline by the wind and attach themselves to small particles of air pollution. When the particles are inhaled, they then have a higher chance of being trapped in the lung because of the static electricity they contain. This means that a greater amount of air pollution may be absorbed into our blood near powerlines compared with away from powerlines.

A large study of the Polish Military over 20 years found increases of between 5 and 14 fold in cases of chronic and acute myeloid leukaemia and Non-Hodgkin's lymphoma when the people became over 50 years of age for personnel who had used radiofrequency and microwave transmitters during their career.

There is contradictory evidence linking mobile phone use and brain tumours and other ill-health complaints. Our analysis of international research concludes that, at present, it is advisable to limit mobile phone use to calls that you consider essential. Text messages are better than talking, but hold the handset away from your body when you press send. Mobile phones work at their highest power (up to 500 times stronger that the rest of the call will use) during the dialling process and the first few seconds of the call – so hold the phone away from your head until the person called actually answers.

Overall, we believe the evidence is that people should avoid unnecessary exposure to EMFs, from electricity pylon lines, transformers, and electrical appliances and they should also avoid using handheld mobile phones more than absolutely essential.

3 What are your risks?

1 Some dangers to health and life are very serious but the risk of actually suffering from them may be very small. These risks can be difficult to work out. It can also be very confusing trying to compare risks.

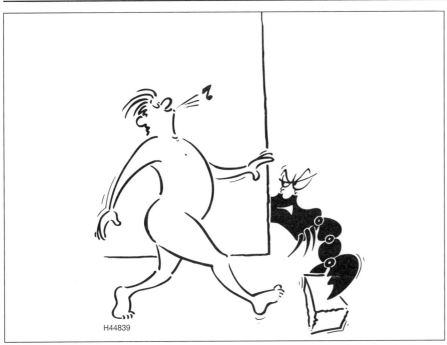

Some dangers to health and life are very serious but the risk of actually suffering from them may be very small

2 For example, the risk of being killed by lightning in the UK is 1 in 10 million. This doesn't mean very much to most of us. So try thinking about it this way.

3 At 1 in 10 million you would need a line of people 10,000 km (6,000 miles) long to contain the single person who would be killed by lightning. It would take 4 months of continuous walking to reach the end.

4 On the other hand, the risk of premature death from smoking 10 cigarettes per day is just over 1 in 100. The line of people would now only be 100 m (100 yards) long and it would only take you 2 minutes to reach the end.

5 Now it starts to make sense!

Reducing risks

6 Some of the risks to health cannot be easily avoided. Many are so small it makes little point even trying to do so.

7 There are some risks, however, which are not only quite high, they are also partly or totally avoidable. Tobacco smoking is a good example. There is a real and significant risk from inhaling other people's smoke (passive smoking) and of course the chances of your health being affected are even greater by actually smoking yourself.

8 So OK, men in the UK have a one in three lifetime chance of developing cancer but of those who get it, three out of four survive! This means the majority survive and go on to live happy, fulfilling and productive lives. Otherwise we would be looking at a very empty country when it came to the male population.

9 Obviously, you can reduce your risk further by following our tips for living more healthily, having regular GP check-ups, and through being more aware of your body and catching symptoms early.

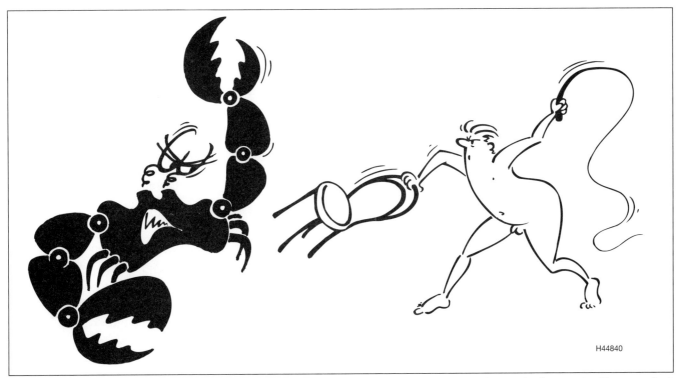

Men in the UK have a one in three lifetime chance of developing cancer but of those who get it, three out of four survive!

Notes

Chapter 2
Routine maintenance (staying healthy)

Contents

1 Obesity and cancer

1 Obesity is the term used when a person's excess weight is enough to cause significantly increased risk of ill health. Obesity leads to a variety of illnesses and conditions, and on average will cause a 9-year reduction in a man's life, commonly because of diabetes, heart disease and stroke.

2 Obesity causes 30,000 deaths in the UK every year, and 18 million working days are lost because of fat-related illness. In America over one third of the population is obese, 300,000 people die each year because of it, and we're following in their footsteps.

3 An obese man is four times as likely to have a heart attack, and can be 30 times more likely to get diabetes, than a

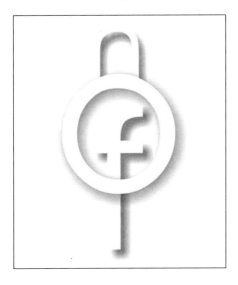

man of normal weight. Obesity also causes arthritis, increases the risk of fatal accidents, asthma, chronic bronchitis, liver disease, kidney disease and depression.

4 Although some overweight men are lucky, and live to a ripe old age without any major problem, most obese men will discover that chronic ill health is in store for them, and the risk is greater the fatter they become. Being fat isn't just a cosmetic problem; it isn't just how you look, it's how you feel, how much energy and life you've got, and how much life you may lose because of illness.

5 As if the above were not enough, being overweight or obese also causes cancer. Nobody would disagree that smoking leads to cancer, but the connection with obesity is less obvious. In fact obesity causes more different types of cancer than smoking, so in some ways it is more dangerous. 1 in 10 cancers are obesity related, and around 1 in 7 of all cancer deaths in the over 50s are caused by obesity, according to a study of nearly 1 million Americans in 2003.

6 Smoking cigarettes causes a large number of cancer deaths, but obesity isn't far behind, and we're set to see an epidemic of weight-related cancers in the next 20 years because of the current epidemic of obesity. The evidence is clear that just as stopping smoking is important if you want to live to see your grandchildren growing up, so is losing weight. The extremely good news is that by losing weight, the extra chances of getting cancer reduce or disappear.

7 There are many different places a

person can store fat – arms, legs, backside – but the place that matters most is the belly. Someone once compared fat people to either apples or pears. 'Pears' are typically women with big rears and thighs, and 'apples' are often men with big bellies. Unfortunately for us, it's the big bellies that are most dangerous, because abdominal fat causes illness. Abdominal fat isn't just under the skin; most of it is inside us, wrapped around our bowels, which means that it's in the place that it can do most harm, doing damage from the inside.

Body mass index (BMI)

8 When you go to see your doctor because you suffer from one of those illnesses, or because you've got a symptom that you think might be serious, he or she may measure your weight and height in order to assess your risk of illness.

9 The calculation based on the relationship between weight and height is called the BMI (Body Mass Index). BMI is calculated as follows:

a) *Using pounds and inches. Multiply your weight in pounds by 700 and divide that figure by the square of your height in inches. For example, if you're 68 inches tall and weigh 185 pounds, your BMI is 185 x 700 ÷ 68 x 68 = 129,500 ÷ 4,624 = 28.*

b) *Using kilograms and metres. Divide your weight in kilograms by the square of your height in metres. This means if you're 1.78 metres tall and weigh 78 kg, your BMI is 78 ÷ 1.78 x 1.78 = 78 ÷ 3.2 = 24.4*

2

Height / weight chart – Imperial (height in inches, weight in pounds)

Height	Underweight	Healthy weight	Overweight	Obese
63	up to 113	113 – 141	141 – 169	169 plus
64	up to115	115 – 144	144 – 173	173 plus
65	up to 121	121 – 151	151 – 182	182 plus
66	up to 124	124 – 155	155 – 186	186 plus
67	up to127	127 – 159	159 – 191	191 plus
68	up to 132	132 – 165	165 – 197	197 plus
69	up to 135	135 – 168	168 – 202	202 plus
70	up to 140	140 – 174	174 – 209	209 plus
71	up to143	143 – 178	178 – 214	214 plus
72	up to 147	147 – 184	184 – 221	221 plus
74	up to 155	155 – 194	194 – 233	233 plus
75	up to 159	159 – 199	199 – 238	238 plus

Height / weight chart – metric (height in metres, weight in kilograms)

Height	Underweight	Healthy weight	Overweight	Obese
1.60	up to 51	51 – 64	64 – 77	77 plus
1.63	up to 52	52 – 65	65 – 79	79 plus
1.65	up to 55	55 – 69	69 – 83	83 plus
1.68	up to 56	56 – 70	70 – 84	84 plus
1.70	up to 58	58 – 72	72 – 87	87 plus
1.73	up to 60	60 – 75	75 – 89	89 plus
1.75	up to 61	61 – 76	76 – 92	92 plus
1.78	up to 64	64 – 79	79 – 95	95 plus
1.80	up to 65	65 – 81	81 – 97	97 plus
1.83	up to 67	67 – 84	84 – 100	100 plus
1.88	up to 70	70 – 88	88 – 106	106 plus
1.91	up to 72	72 – 90	90 – 108	108 plus

10 The higher your BMI gets, the fatter you are, and the higher your risk of illness. If your BMI is 30 or above, you are technically obese. This is an emotive word, but is used with great care, because it means that you're fat enough to become ill, and possibly die early because of your weight.

11 Another, easier way to assess your risk is to measure your waist circumference with a tape, positioning the tape midway between the bottom ribs at the side and the crest of your hip and resting 1 cm below the belly-button; if you are 102 cm (4 in) or more, then you are at significantly increased risk.

How does obesity cause cancer?

12 Obesity causes a number of different illnesses, including cancer, in a number of different ways which are not yet fully understood. What we do know is that fat people don't deal with sugar very well.

13 Muscles use sugar for fuel; our 'fuel

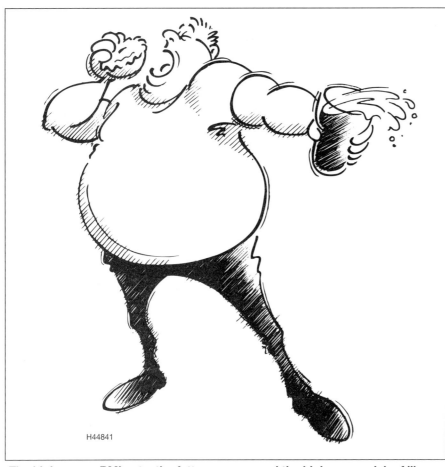

H44841

The higher your BMI gets, the fatter you are, and the higher your risk of illness

tank' is the blood stream where sugar circulates before being used, and when we run out of sugar we don't function well, so we fill the tank up by eating. Sugar doesn't just come from sweet stuff, our bodies also extract sugar from carbohydrates such as bread and pasta, to prevent the needle going onto 'empty'.

14 The muscles use a hormone called insulin, made in the pancreas, to extract the sugar from the blood. The more sugar we have, the more insulin we need. Fat people have too much sugar in the blood and an increased resistance to the effects of insulin, so they need to overproduce insulin to deliver enough sugar to the muscles. They end up having not only too much sugar, but also too much insulin. The excess sugar can lead to diabetes, and the extra insulin has serious damaging effects of its own.

15 Insulin is a dangerous substance if you have too much of it. When it circulates in the blood, all the tissues of

the body come into contact with it, and its toxic effects. Each tissue or organ of the body reacts in a different way to insulin: the kidneys retain too much salt in the blood, putting blood pressure up; the glands produce abnormal hormones, affecting sex drive and fertility; other organs such as the bowel react by becoming inflamed, and eventually developing cancer.

16 So by being fat, a man poisons himself, and the poison is made *within* the body, every minute of every day.

Toxic waist

17 There's even more bad news. Fatty tissue doesn't just sit buried inside our abdomens doing nothing. Instead it acts like a lump of toxic waste buried in concrete in our countryside; it leaks hazardous chemicals into the water supply and wreaks havoc. These hazardous chemicals, one in particular called IGF-1, mixed together with insulin, are called 'Fat Toxins'.

Cancer of the bowel

18 Cancer of the bowel is the third most common cancer in America, and one of the cancers most closely linked with obesity. Weight related bowel cancers usually occur in the large bowel or colon, at the far end of the gut, where the last part of the digestive process occurs, but can occur elsewhere in the bowel. Although related to obesity, cancer of the colon may cause unexplained weight *loss*, as well as a change in bowel habit, or sometimes the passage of blood or mucus with a motion. See Chapter 6 for more details.

19 Obesity causes colon cancer in two ways. One is the action of fat toxins on the cells of the bowel. The cells lining the gut are naturally lost and replaced very quickly, and such rapidly growing cells are susceptible to cancer-causing chemicals, like fat toxins. The other reason seems to be that some cancer-causing chemicals within our food are absorbed by fatty tissue, and trapped for a long time; because obese men store more fat, they store more of these carcinogens, leading to bowel cancer.

Cancer of the prostate and testicular cancer

20 Cancers of the prostate gland and testicles have strong links with obesity. Prostate cancer is more common the older we get, and the fatter we get, so we're all at risk. Because of the increasing levels of obesity in the population, what we're currently seeing is just the tip of the iceberg of obesity-related cancers, before a huge increase in cases of bowel and prostate cancer occurs in the next few years. An enlarged prostate may cause the flow of urine to be weak, and slow to start and stop. Sufferers may have to get up at night to pass water, and go more frequently during the day. Although most cases of enlarged prostate are *not* because of cancer, the symptoms are similar. See Chapter 7.

21 Fat toxins are partly to blame for cancer of the prostate, but obesity also has an effect on male hormones which are also involved in tumour formation. The normal levels of hormones like testosterone, which keep us healthy, energetic, and maintain our sex drive, are disturbed by obesity. Fat tissue behaves like a sponge when hormones

2

are around, so the more fat we have, the more hormone is soaked up from the blood, and the less we have left to give us sex drive and energy. Once inside the fatty sponge, a chemical reaction occurs, altering the character of the hormone before it finds its way back into the blood, and it's these altered, abnormal hormone levels which can have devastating effects.

22 In fact, because of this reaction men actually end up having raised levels of oestrogen, the female sex hormone. The result can be erectile dysfunction and impotence, or reduced fertility, making it difficult for a man to have sex and for a couple to have children. Being fat can not only make your genitals difficult to find, but once you've located them, they may not work!

23 In women, similar hormone problems resulting from obesity can have even worse effects, causing abnormalities of the ovaries, and a big increase in the risk of breast cancer, and cancer of the womb. But for men, the risk is of prostate cancer and testicular cancer.

24 Two large American studies in 2003 found that obese men, with a body mass index of 30 or more, had more aggressive forms of prostate cancer and were 60% more likely to get a recurrence after treatment than men of normal weight. The studies recommended that sufferers of the disease should lose weight to increase their chance of survival.

Cancer of the liver

25 When a person is obese he has too much fat inside the abdomen, which surrounds and wraps the internal organs, including the gut, even extending up to the heart. But the fat also turns up *inside* the liver. More often than not the liver manages to carry on doing its job despite the extra fat, but sometimes the fat causes the liver to malfunction in the same way as drinking too much alcohol does. In severe cases, as with alcohol, this leads to cirrhosis, liver failure, jaundice and sometimes liver cancer. The risks are much greater if a person is both obese and a heavy drinker. Abnormalities in the liver can be picked up on blood tests, or on ultrasound examination.

26 Obesity is also linked with gallstones and gall-bladder cancer.

Cancer of the kidney

27 One cause of cancer of the kidney, or renal cell carcinoma, is the circulating fat toxins in obese people. The kidneys are extremely sensitive to these toxins, and also respond by retaining salt in the body, instead of removing it in the urine. This causes high blood pressure in the same way as eating too much salty food, so obese people in particular should limit the amount of salt they eat.

Cancer of the oesophagus and stomach

28 Cancer of the oesophagus causes difficulty in swallowing food, and can eventually block the food pipe altogether – see Chapter 6. Various different things make oesophageal cancer more likely, including drinking spirits, smoking, and heavily spiced food, but obesity has a role to play as well.

29 The lining of the oesophagus is sensitive. It is protected from the strong acid produced by the stomach by a valve which opens and shuts to let food through. The oesophagus should only come into contact with the food we eat, and saliva. In obesity, the bulk of the fat around the abdomen actually squashes the stomach, forcing the contents up through the closed valve and into the foodpipe. This will initially cause symptoms of indigestion and heartburn, but if persistent and prolonged can lead to cancer.

30 The top of the stomach, or cardia, is also at risk of cancer because of the abnormal flow of acid. An obese person who also smokes or drinks spirits has a much greater risk.

Other cancers

31 The more that scientists come to understand the disease, the more fat toxins in the blood are being blamed for different cancers. The list of cancers linked to obesity now also include the pancreas, small bowel, throat, lymphoma, Hodgkin's disease, and gall-bladder cancer.

Other risks

32 As well as actually being responsible for some cancers, obesity acts as an obstacle in the fight against cancer at every step of the way, whether or not a particular tumour is caused by obesity:

- It makes it more difficult for a person to discover the early signs of cancer; it's harder to find a lump if its hidden by surplus flesh.
- The symptoms of cancer may be masked by symptoms of obesity; breathlessness due to a lung tumour may be mistaken for unfitness because of overweight, or bone pain may be put down to aching joints or arthritis, when it may be because of a bony tumour.
- It is more difficult for the doctor to perform a thorough examination and pick up subtle signs of cancer when hampered by a pillow of fat. Signs such as enlargement of the liver or a lump in the bowel could be missed and allow the disease to get worse and spread.
- X-rays, ultrasounds or other tests may be less accurate in an obese person, because the image may be blurred in the presence of too much fat.
- Any operation needed to diagnose or remove a malignant growth will be far more complex and less likely to succeed in an obese patient. The operation will take longer, be technically more challenging, and there will be more blood lost. The anaesthetist will have to use more gas, and will have to be careful to prevent complications of breathing including pulmonary embolism and infection. The recovery after surgery is more hazardous, and there is risk of pressure sores, deep vein thrombosis (DVT) and wound infection. It is harder for nurses and families to care for an obese person without risking back injuries through lifting.
- It can be difficult to work out and apply the correct doses of anti-cancer drugs in obese people because fatty tissue absorbs some drugs like a sponge, making them less effective.

How can the risk of obesity-related cancer be reduced?

33 The risk of obesity-related cancer can only be significantly reduced by losing weight, but the good news is that by losing 10% of his weight, a man can *halve* his risk of dying from these diseases. It is usually unrealistic to try and get to the same weight 'as when you were 18' or your 'ideal weight', but studies show that a relatively small reduction in weight, if maintained, has major health benefits.

34 As well as varying lifestyle in order to lose weight there are specific dietary and exercise recommendations relating to cancer risk. A wide variety of fruit and vegetables should be consumed to help protect against cancer, because a low intake seems to increase risk, especially of bowel and stomach cancer. Additional fibre should be included in the diet to lower the risk of colon and pancreatic cancer, but a large intake of red meat may exaggerate the risk, so some experts suggest it should be limited. Diet should be low in saturated fat.

35 High levels of physical activity are known to provide some protection against colon cancer. The International Agency for Research on Cancer suggest that 13–14% of cases of colon cancer are attributable to a sedentary lifestyle, although some studies suggest a 70% reduction in cases of colon cancer in active individuals.

36 For protection against cancer, any exercise will do as long as enough energy is expended, so a short burst of vigorous exercise has as much benefit as prolonged moderate exercise. For the purposes of weight loss, however, exercise should be brisk rather than vigorous, and in any case should be maintained as a permanent way of life.

37 Women who are physically active have a substantial reduction in risk of breast cancer, so exercise as a family benefits everyone. There is also some evidence that physical activity helps to protect against prostate cancer, but research is still being done; the likelihood is that the reduction in the risk is only moderate.

How to lose weight

38 Obesity is caused by taking in more energy as food than is burned off by activity. Some people seem to eat less than others and still gain weight, others can eat non-stop, and not gain an ounce, but that is just a fact of life. Another fact of life is that if you're obese you probably need to eat less and do more.

You Are What You Eat

39 Sometimes the answer is just to cut down on food, by reducing portion sizes, and trying to avoid snacks between meals; but sometimes the type of food has to change. It is important to have a well-balanced diet, containing protein, carbohydrate, and a certain amount of fat, but not too much.

40 As a general rule, the sort of food that is high in fat and bad for us is the sort of food that *looks* bad for us, i.e. it's fairly obvious. Chips, crisps, fry-ups, pies, fatty meat, junk food, many takeaways and chocolate are good examples. Foods like this should only be eaten as occasional treats, because they contain saturated fats, and are very high in calories, which cause weight gain.

41 There's plenty of enjoyable food that is healthy and can be eaten without guilt. Curries and stir-fries can be extremely healthy without spoiling their appeal; meat and fish, fruit, bread and pasta, can be eaten freely, as long as they're prepared healthily (which is just as easy as preparing them unhealthily).

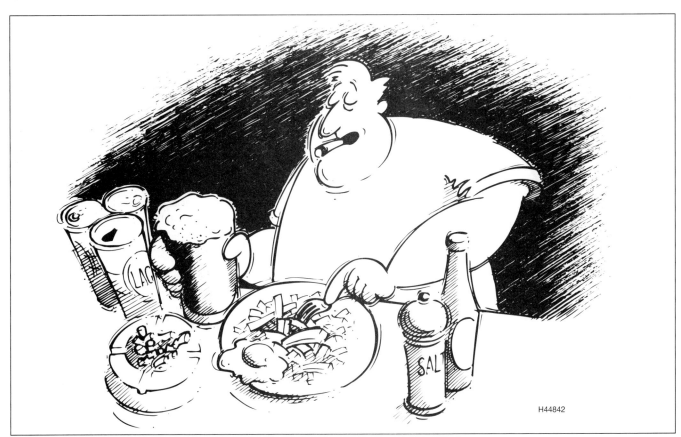

H44842

The sort of food that is high in fat and bad for us is the sort of food that *looks* bad for us

'You Should Get Out More!'

42 Physical activity is essential in the fight against obesity and against cancer in particular. It also protects against high blood pressure, high cholesterol and heart disease, so if you have a sitting-down job, watch too much TV, or drive short journeys instead of walking, you need to have a rethink.

43 Physical activity can be increased as part of the daily routine without going down to the local gym, although sport and swimming are beneficial. The ideal intensity of exercise to lose weight is brisk enough for you to be breathless, and work up a sweat, but without preventing you from talking. Brisk walking fits the bill; try walking up the stairs or escalators instead of using the lift. Walk to work instead of using the bus, or walk a couple of blocks to buy a (healthy) lunch; never use the car for short journeys like buying a newspaper.

44 Gardening is a great way to take some exercise. Even housework counts, but that might be taking things too far! Any exercise helps, even something as simple as standing up when using the telephone. Switch the TV off at meal times; you will eat more slowly, therefore less quantity, you'll talk and gesticulate more, and shuffle your knife and fork round, which all use energy.

45 To stay healthy, a man should do at least 30 minutes of exercise every day, in one spell or in combination, but a man needing to lose weight, or avoid regaining weight already lost, must do as much as possible, even 60–90 minutes per day.

46 If you start doing unaccustomed exercise you should do it carefully until you get into the swing of it, and you shouldn't expect to lose a lot of weight initially by exercise alone, as some fat will convert into muscle, which is actually heavier than fat! You will probably find that your waist circumference reduces and your clothes become looser, which are excellent signs that you're winning the battle.

Next year's model

47 If the prevalence of obesity increases at the current rate, we may not notice much difference from one day to the next, or even from one year to the next, but there's no doubt that we'll see the disastrous effects of obesity in the next generation. Our children's health will be wrecked by obesity, diabetes, heart disease and cancer. We need to reduce our own *personal* chances of getting diseases, including cancer, by becoming more aware of our weight, what we eat, and what activity we do. But we also need to ensure that our children follow suit, even though they may be too young to make the correct choices themselves, because unless we take a very serious view of our children's way of living, we'll find that they are dying before we do, and it will be our fault.

How to get help

48 If your efforts at losing weight are unsuccessful, there are many ways of seeking help. Many slimming clubs like Rosemary Conley, Weight Watchers and Slimming World will accept men, although men are sometimes reluctant to enrol. Internet websites which teach manageable lifestyle change are an alternative, and can often provide invaluable assistance. There are shelves crammed with books on weight loss in any shop, but they can be misleading, and choosing the correct one can be a nightmare.

49 If none of these appeal, or if they don't work, go to your local GP surgery where your practice nurse or doctor will help. They may provide information and encouragement or refer you to a dietician, but if necessary there are safe and effective weight loss medications which your GP can prescribe.

50 Help and counselling by a therapist is useful for some people, others may need

H44864

Physical activity protects against high blood pressure, high cholesterol and heart disease

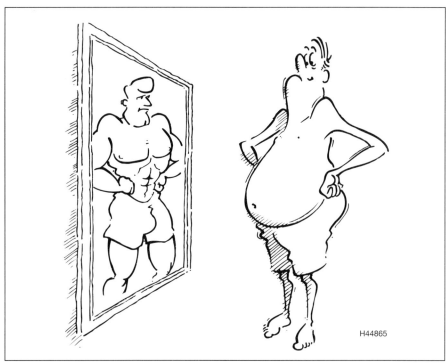

Many slimming clubs will accept men, although men are sometimes reluctant to enrol

referring to a hospital specialist, or even be advised to undergo an operation, which nowadays is done by keyhole surgery. Many pharmacists now provide weight loss advice.

Further information

51 If you would like to know more, look at the contacts section at the back of this book, or contact: www.fatmanslim.com

2 Occupational cancer

Introduction

1 Workers may rightly be concerned that exposure to something at work could cause cancer. The mechanism by which this can happen is complex, and where it does arise cancers may not actually appear until many decades later (typically 20–30 years) – sometimes long after the worker has left the work that resulted in the exposure.

2 Occupational cancers are those that arise after exposure to a physical, chemical or biological substance in the workplace. Less than one in ten of all cancers occur this way, although in some

cases a workplace exposure can work with another risk factor (such as smoking) to increase the risk of cancer occurring – for example asbestos workers who smoke may be ten times as likely to get lung cancer as those who don't.

3 Occupational cancers tend to occur at younger ages than those arising from other causes.

4 In the UK about 6,000 cancer deaths a year are attributed to occupational cancer.

History

5 Percival Pott is credited with describing the first well-known occupational cancer – when he noted that many "climbing boy" chimney sweeps developed cancer of the scrotum, from contact with soot.

6 In the 1820s workers with a chemical called arsenic were often found to develop skin cancer (as indeed did those who used cosmetics containing arsenic!). During the Industrial Revolution workers suddenly found that their work brought them in to contact with oils, pitch, tar, soot and other noxious mixtures – many workers developed skin cancer and for some occupations it was simply accepted that the job was dangerous and you would die early.

7 Workers in dye factories, gas works, chemical industries and the rubber industry became known to be at risk for particular cancers. Metal miners often developed lung cancer, dye workers developed bladder cancer and later still experiments with X-ray radiation produced cancers from which some of the early pioneers died.

8 In 1939 the link between making PVC (poly vinyl chloride) and a rare cancer of the liver was recognised. Later still, a clever piece of research in the rubber industry identified the chemical that was causing a group of workers to develop bladder cancer. 'Carcinogen' became the word used to describe something that could cause cancer.

9 Over the years many different occupations and many different agents have been identified with the potential to be associated with cancer – the list is long and often the link has only became clear many decades later (for instance, a linkage between nasal cancer and furniture making was long suspected, but unproven – hardwood dusts are now known to be the risk factor).

10 Today many hazards are known, and two important priorities exist:
- Making work safe, ensuring that workers don't get exposed to things that have a risk of causing cancer.
- Ensuring that those who develop cancer get early diagnosis and treatment, and that where appropriate an occupational cause is investigated to ensure other workers aren't at risk for the future.

Recognising occupational cancer

11 This can be difficult as the cancer often comes many years after the original contact – proving a link can be complex and is made even more difficult as lifestyle and other risk factors, even exposure to chemicals at home (hobbies being an important and often neglected area) may act as additional risk factors.

12 Recognising a group of cases in a number of people doing similar work with a similar type of cancer has been the commonest way of suspecting an occupational cause. It is this technique, known as epidemiology, which has identified the occupations and hazards described above.

2

13 Other well-known examples are:
- Lung cancer or mesothelioma (a cancer of the lung covering) after exposure to asbestos – shipyard workers were particularly at risk in the past.
- Nasal cancer after contact with nickel compounds or hardwood dusts – furniture makers and miners were at risk.
- Leukaemia or other cancers involving the blood arising after contact with benzene – petroleum workers.
- Skin cancer after exposure to ultraviolet radiation (including the sun!) or exposure to pitch or tars – outdoor workers may be at risk.
- Bladder cancer from exposure to certain chemicals – rubber industry workers were at risk.

14 As already written – many and various cancers can occur, and many and various agents may cause them.

15 Suspected carcinogens are carefully investigated. Laws now exist to prevent workers being exposed to risks and known carcinogens are usually banned, or can only be used in a workplace with suitable precautions.

16 Where workers are known to be at risk – perhaps because of a risk that occurred in the past, which has now been recognised to be a cancer causing one – monitoring and screening can be used to ensure that any symptoms or signs of cancers developing are found promptly. Early diagnosis and treatment, just as with cancers not related to occupation, are important.

17 Workers who may be at risk are usually told to see their doctor if they have unusual symptoms, a cough, finding blood where it shouldn't be or signs specific to the cancer risk involved.

18 Questionnaires can be used regularly – asking about symptoms like cough or skin disease (often used in paint sprayers and mechanics to enable early detection of symptoms of occupational disease – not just cancer). If symptoms are found then tests can be done to establish whether a serious health problem exists or not (not every cough is cancer!).

19 In some occupations with a known risk, regular tests or screening are done – this can be a simple urine test, a medical examination, a blood test or a lung test for example.

20 Detection is obviously important – but prevention is better!

Preventing occupational cancer

21 In very simple terms, if something is known to cause cancer – then avoiding it is the best way of not getting the cancer (this is like the statement in a previous British Army Manual … the best way of avoiding being killed by a nuclear bomb is not to be there when it goes off …).

22 If a carcinogen is known, then stopping its use, its presence or its manufacture in the workplace is the best way of getting rid of the risk. (Let's take the analogy of being a gladiator in a sword fight – if you take away the swords it is much harder to get hurt!)

23 Substitution – using a different chemical or agent to do the same job – is one way of avoiding the use of a known risky substance. (Substituting a feather duster for a sword obviously helps to reduce injuries in the sword fight!)

24 If it can't be got rid of completely, then reducing the amount needed can help to reduce the risks of a worker being harmed. (This is like cutting the end off the sword, so our warrior is less likely to get hit by it – and if he does get hit, perhaps it causes less damage.)

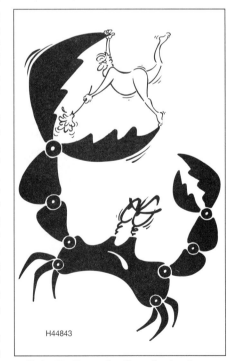

H44843

Substituting a feather duster for a sword obviously helps to reduce injuries in the sword fight!

25 However, for some chemicals, contact with even very small quantities is dangerous and, with a risk of cancer, complete avoidance is preferable. (Remember the British Army and the nuclear bomb!)

26 Workplaces can be changed to reduce contact between people and the known risk – machinery, processes and work tasks can be changed to ensure no contact is possible between the nasty agent and the worker. (Continuing the sword fight analogy – in this scenario you put the other fighter with a sword in a different room, or in a barred cage.)

27 As a last resort (as other methods are better) protective clothing such as gloves, masks or even breathing apparatus can be used to avoid contact between the worker and the substance concerned. (Here our fighter wears armour to reduce the likelihood of injury … but the tricky bit is to ensure the armour is of the right type, fits well and has no "chinks".)

28 Care is needed, however – cancers have occurred when protective clothing, pockets or gloves have become so contaminated with the chemical they were designed to protect against that they have increased rather than decreased the exposure of the worker.

29 Safe ways of working, including safe ways of disposing or cleaning protective equipment, are vital. Some workplaces have pre-employment health screening, but in practice it is rarely effective to identify and exclude workers who themselves may be at risk. (This could be thought of as trying to select the fittest fighter you can – but fortunately even a less fit swordsman can fight without being hurt if he is well-trained and well-equipped – give him a rifle and he will still win.)

30 Above all – where known risks exist workers need to know about them. They have a right to information about the potential risks they work with and can be also told what to look out for. Knowing about a workplace risk can make it more likely that a safe way of working is followed – and one worker can help to keep a colleague safe. (In simple terms this is telling your gladiator that the sword is sharp and teaching him how to avoid the point.)

31 Information should be given encouraging workers to see a doctor or a nurse, or report symptoms to a manager, and at the same time known additional risks can be explained and avoided. Stopping or reducing smoking for example can make a big difference to the risk of developing lung cancer – occupational or non-occupational. Avoiding over-exposure to the sun, by being burnt to a frazzle on holiday, may reduce the chances of skin cancer arising. A healthy diet can reduce risk for many cancers and a generally healthy lifestyle is no bad thing. (Here our swordsman is being encouraged not to eat a heavy meal or get drunk before he steps in to the arena!)

32 Finally – workers themselves have an important role in prevention, firstly in terms of using and following safe ways to work. As a swordsman given a winning battle plan you are daft not to use it. And secondly if a worker is suspicious about something being a risk that is not properly controlled – ask! (The gladiator spots an unguarded sword and asks whether someone may get hurt.)

What to do if you think you have occupational cancer

33 Don't ignore it! Many workers, especially men, tend to think that medical problems will go away on their own and prefer to avoid the hassle of seeking advice or treatment. This is a mistake. Early advice is best – don't be afraid to ask.

34 Ask advice from an experienced colleague or a manager – if a known risk exists they will probably be able to tell you where to go for help. You don't need to share the details of what is actually hurting or worrying you – simply say that things aren't right and seek advice about where to get help.

35 Many employers have occupational health departments. These employ doctors and nurses who are familiar with the workplace risks and who can provide advice or organise any testing that may be necessary.

36 Alternatively see a doctor or ring the NHS Helpline – but if you are worried that your symptoms may be caused by something at work, don't forget to ensure you mention this in the conversation. (It is often forgotten, and not always asked for.) Doctors and nurses are used to talking about odd things happening to bodies – don't be

embarrassed, tell them what you are worried about.

37 Don't be worried if further tests are needed. Many symptoms are not caused by cancer, but tests are needed to give you the right advice or treatment.

38 If a medical problem is confirmed – then there may be a need to test the workplace or other workers to ensure that the risk involved doesn't continue or injure others.

39 Occupational cancer is a reportable disease; regulatory authorities may investigate the workplace to ensure hazards and risks are adequately-controlled. Employers in the UK have a duty to report cases of occupational disease, under legislation known as RIDDOR (Reporting of Injuries, Diseases and Dangerous Occurrences).

40 Industrial injuries disablement benefit is claimable in the UK for some types of cancer – usually those with a well-established occupational link (such as bladder cancer and exposure to beta-naphthylamine, nasal cancer and hardwood dust exposure, etc) and information about eligibility should be obtained.

41 If an employer has been negligent in failing to control a well-known risk then compensation can be sought via the civil

courts, although proving cause and effect is often hard.

42 The Health & Safety Executive is a good source of advice with much information available on request (see *Contacts*), as also do Trade Unions if available.

3 Prevention

World Cancer
Research Fund

Introduction

1 You've probably heard the statistic: one in four of us is likely to develop cancer at some time in our life. But research shows that there are convincing links between the food and lifestyle choices you make and your risk of cancer. Cancer can take 20 years or more to develop. So, although it's never too late to start, the sooner you begin on a healthier path, the better your chances.

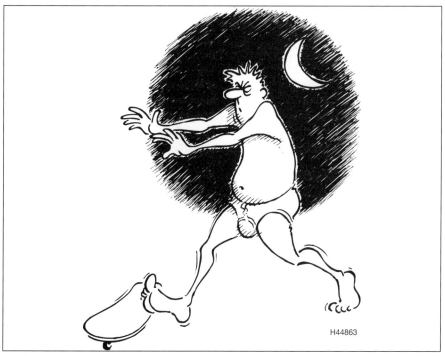

Although it's never too late to start, the sooner you begin on a healthier path, the better your chances

Scientists now believe that as many as 30 to 40 per cent of new cancer cases could be prevented by making healthier food and lifestyle choices.

What causes cancer?

2 Cancer begins when the genetic information in a single cell becomes damaged in some way and causes it to divide at an uncontrolled rate. The resulting group of cells often forms a lump or swelling – which is usually referred to as a 'tumour'. The tumour may then grow and go on to damage surrounding healthy tissues or organs, or cancer cells may break away from the original tumour and spread through the bloodstream or the lymphatic system to other parts of the body – a process known as 'metastasis'.

Is it mainly inherited?

3 Inheritance does play a role but we now know that it is the environmental factors – including diet and lifestyle – that have the strongest influence on whether we develop cancer or not. In fact, when more than one family member develops cancer it's more likely to be due to chance, or shared lifestyle, than to inherited genetic factors. Only 5 to 10 per cent of cancer cases are attributed to the presence of an inherited gene mutation ('cancer gene'). This is good

news because it means there is something we can do about it. In fact, the greatest hope in the fight against cancer lies in prevention.

Migrant studies

4 Migrant studies were some of the first to suggest that environment was responsible for the large differences in cancer rates across different regions and countries. People migrating from one county to another (with a different pattern of cancers) will, within one or two generations, have much the same pattern of cancers as current inhabitants.
5 For instance, some studies show that rates of stomach cancer decreased among Chinese men as they moved from Shanghai to the USA. Rates of this cancer were shown to be four to six times higher in Shanghai compared with the USA – this can largely be explained by the high salt diets in China. Likewise, prostate cancer incidence among these men increased 10-15 times. Since diet and lifestyle make up the major differences between these countries, this reinforces the concept that cancer can be prevented.

What can you do?

6 Although there are no guarantees, there are positive steps you can take to reduce your risk of cancer and other serious disease. Besides not smoking and cutting down on booze, there are other aspects of your diet and lifestyle that you'll need to tackle.

7 There are some foods that may actually help to prevent, or slow down, the cancer process. Recent scientific evidence shows that eating a diet rich in vegetables and fruits can prevent one in five cases – and possibly more – of all cancers. So it's a case of more of these foods, and less of the junk.

Start with some investigation

8 It's wise to ask your relatives about the types of cancers (if any) that run in your family.
9 If one (or both) of your parents have suffered from a particular cancer at an early age (i.e., before 50 or so), then it's important that you find out what you can do to protect yourself against that particular disease. Of course, there are no absolute guarantees against developing cancer but, just like heart disease, there are lots of positive things we can do – starting right now.

Beware of media stories

10 Flick through any tabloid newspaper or glossy magazine and you'll be bombarded with sensational stories about diet and health. And, in any one publication over the space of a few weeks, it's not unusual to read entirely conflicting advice. If your health wasn't such a serious business it might be vaguely amusing. But sometimes the health information that's offered is false or misleading. It's amazing how many 'one-off' research studies are printed which convince the public that 'everything gives you cancer'.
11 Don't be rattled. Take a step back and adopt some healthy scepticism. What really matters in all things to do with health, is the overall scientific evidence. But the fact of the matter is that 'sensible' balanced stories just don't sell newspapers. So, when you encounter sensational health stories about 'proven' cancer causes in newspapers, magazines, television shows, radio programmes or on the Internet, use your common sense. Make sure the information is science-based and the source is reliable. Remember that research studies show that the major factors in cancer risk are things that are in your control.

Making changes

12 Before you begin, it's important to be honest about how willing you are to

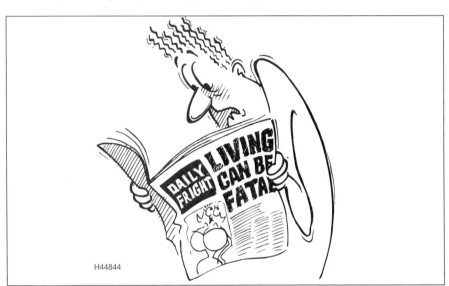

H44844

Flick through any tabloid newspaper and you'll be bombarded with sensational stories about diet and health

make changes to your diet and lifestyle. Most of us tend not to like changes and it's true that it's not always easy. But remind yourself that changes that seem awkward at first will become more comfortable as you practice them. Remember learning to drive? You'll recall that the initial difficulty eventually faded with practice and persistence. The same applies to developing new, healthier habits. Just like driving a car, with time, it'll become almost automatic.

13 The changes which you need to make will obviously depend on what your lifestyle is like now. Not everybody will be starting from the same point so it is important to look at the type of life you lead now, as a whole, and assess how it relates to the lifestyle recommended for cancer prevention.

Obstacles

14 Before changing your habits, it's important to think about, and prepare for, any obstacles that might interfere with your success. On a blank page, write down the obstacles that you think you may face when trying to achieve your goals. Finally, add in the ways in which you think you can overcome these. For example, an obstacle to giving up smoking is that you always associate smoking with having a drink. One way around this is simply to avoid the pub for a few weeks or months.

Following a few simple dietary and lifestyle guidelines, such as maintaining a healthy body weight, could prevent up to 100,000 cases of cancer in the UK, and 3 to 4 million worldwide, every year.

Think about it

15 The very first step is to think about your reasons for wanting to become healthier. An example is, 'my father developed cancer, so I want to take steps now to avoid my chances of getting it in the future' or 'I've recently turned 40 and I need to start taking more care of myself'.

Set out your goals

16 Next, set down your specific goals. It's important to be realistic. Try not to tackle too many changes at once. Just list the goals that are most important to you. The others can follow later. Here are just a few examples to start thinking about:
- Eat a healthier diet.
- Give up smoking – once and for all.
- Lose weight – and keep it off.
- Cut down on alcohol.
- Be more physically active.

17 Write down your specific goals. Make sure that they are realistic and achievable. Underneath, add in how you think making these changes would improve your life. Reading this list once a week, or in moments of weakness, will motivate you to keep going. For example, your goal could be 'Eat a healthier diet' and the corresponding benefits could be, 'This will improve my overall health and give me the energy I need for my stressful job'.

18 The food and lifestyle habits that you have developed are likely to be ingrained from many years of use. But that doesn't mean you can't make changes. Start by thinking about actions you'll need to take in order to change your habits. For instance, if you intend to give up smoking, you could start by setting a date to give up. Next up, you could talk to your GP about trying some nicotine replacement products.

19 The important thing is to take it slowly. Develop a pace that works for you – one that you are likely to stick with. This is not about punishment or self-denial. It's about treating your body well and making your health a priority.

Put the right fuel in

20 Traditionally, meals are often planned around meat. Vegetables and other foods that come from plants (such as rice, pasta, bread or beans) are then often added as an accompaniment. But did you know that changing the focus of your meals is actually one of the best ways to improve your health? Swap it around. Instead of focusing on the meat you'll have, make plant foods the main part of your meal. Aim to fill two thirds or more of your plate with these nutritious foods. And try to think of animal foods (that is, the meat, fish or low fat dairy products) as the accompaniment to your meal. These foods should fill the remaining part of your plate – that is, one third or less.

Plant foods are foods that come from plants – such as vegetables, fruits or grains – rather than from animals. These include: cereals such as grains, bread, rice and pasta; tubers such as potatoes, sweet potatoes and yams; vegetables and fruits such as fresh or frozen green vegetables, root vegetables, salad vegetables, vegetable/fruit juice and canned, dried or fresh fruit; pulses such as beans, peas and lentils; nuts and seeds such as brazil nuts, cashew nuts, pumpkin seeds and sesame seeds.

2

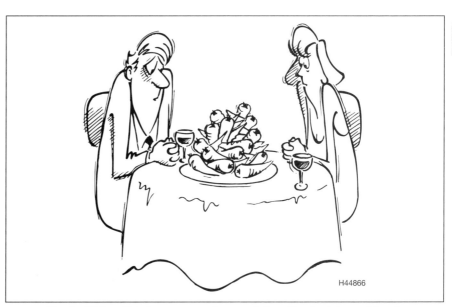

H44866

Aim to fill two thirds or more of your plate with plant-based foods

Animal foods are those foods that come from animals such as chickens, lambs, pigs or cows. These foods include: meat, game, eggs, cheese, milk, poultry and fish.

What's the easy way?

- Aim to have a colourful salad with lunch or dinner – or a side salad when eating out.
- Add beans or lentils to salads, stews, soups or pasta/rice dishes. Try different kinds, such as yellow lentils, chick peas, cannellini, kidney, pinto or black beans.
- Make salads and soups into tasty main dishes by adding some reduced fat cheese, beans or a handful of seeds such as pumpkin or sesame seeds sprinkled on top.
- Make a huge bowl of fruit salad for a healthy start to the day. Keep it in the fridge, ready for breakfast (have with yoghurt and cereal), as a healthy dessert or even just to snack on during the day.
- Buy fresh vegetable soup to have handy when you want something quick and tasty, but healthy at the same time.

Meal makeover

21 Below is a good example of how changing the proportions of foods on your plate can make a big difference. The healthier version is much lower in fat and salt, and higher in vitamins, so it would definitely be the better option for your health. It will get you well on your way to achieving the recommended five or more portions of vegetables and fruits each day.

Natural or pill form?

22 Would you consider taking vitamin pills in the hope that they'd offset unhealthy living or a poor diet? Although there is no harm in taking a 'regular' multi-vitamin or mineral tablet – one which does not exceed the daily reference nutrient intake – there is a real lack of evidence to show that many of these pills are actually beneficial for health at all. And so far there is little or no evidence to show they help reduce cancer risk.

23 There are cases where taking vitamin pills may be necessary. For instance, some people can't get all the necessary nutrients from their diet, perhaps because they are not eating enough. Others, such as the elderly, may not be able to absorb vitamins or minerals from their diet so well. If you suspect that you may fall into one or more of these groups, talk to your GP or a qualified dietician.

24 So, before you reach for your usual stash of dietary supplements, stop and think. If you are relatively healthy, with access to a wide variety of healthy foods, there should be no need for them.

25 Experts advise that we eat five or more portions of different vegetables and fruits each day. But surveys show that, unfortunately, most of us aren't reaching that target. So, instead of relying on vitamin pills, just aim to double your intake of vegetables and fruits – this is the best way of getting the nutrients your body needs. These nutrients include vitamins, minerals, fibre and 'phytochemicals', substances that have been proven to help prevent cancer.

How much again?

26 Below are some examples of what a portion of vegetables and fruits looks

like. But this is just a guide. Try not to get too hung up on measurements – you just need to eat a 'decent' sized serving. The overall aim is to double your daily intake – everybody has a different starting point.

Research shows that if we all ate the recommended five or more portions of vegetables and fruits every day, overall cancer rates could be reduced by about 20%. Despite this, 53% of UK people we asked were not aware that their diet could influence their risk of cancer.

One portion of vegetables is equal to:
2-3 heaped tablespoons of most vegetables (like spinach, carrots, peas or sweetcorn).
2 heaped tablespoons of beans (like baked beans or kidney beans).
1 cereal bowlful of salad (like lettuce, tomato and onion).

One portion of fruit is equal to:
1 large slice of large melon or pineapple.
1 whole apple or banana.
2 whole plums or satsumas.
1 handful of raspberries or grapes.
1 glass (150ml) of fresh fruit juice like orange or tomato.
Fruit juice and beans each count only once towards your 5+ a day total – no matter how much of them you drink or eat. And remember, although potatoes are a healthy component of a balanced diet, they cannot be counted in your 5+ total.

Tips to fit in 5+ a day

27 Many people ask 'how can I fit in 5+ portions of vegetables and fruits each

Traditional breakfast brunch	Healthier version
2 rashers back bacon, grilled	2 rashers of reduced salt back bacon, fat trimmed and grilled
2 fried eggs	1 poached egg
2 grilled sausages	small tin baked beans
1 slice fried white bread	grilled mushrooms
Tomato ketchup	grilled tomatoes with chopped basil
	1 slice wholemeal toast with scraping of low fat spread
	1 glass fresh orange juice
This breakfast provides 850 calories, 60 grams fat, 2.63 grams sodium and just a trace of fibre and vitamin C.	This healthier version provides 488 calories, 15 grams fat, 1.62 grams sodium, 11 grams fibre and 80mg vitamin C.

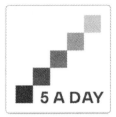

Just Eat More
(fruit & veg)

day?' Here's how it can be done (choose a few each day to make up 5 or more):

Breakfast
Glass of fruit juice.
Fruit salad with yoghurt.
Chopped fresh or dried fruit on cereal.

Snack
Handful of dried fruit.
Piece of fresh fruit.
Vegetable crudités with salsa or hummus.

Lunch
Baked beans on toast.
Home-made vegetable soup.
Large green/side salad.
Sandwich with extra salad.

Dinner
Vegetable stir-fry or curry.
Ratatouille with poultry, fish or lean meat.
Extra vegetables with your main course.
Fresh fruit with dessert.

Fat facts

28 In the UK, many people eat too much fat – probably due to the fact that we're always rushing about and eating 'on the go'. But there is a cost to this: our health. We know that by cutting down on fat we could improve our overall health – so why don't we? The fact is that many of the foods we find most appealing are high in fat. It gives food a certain flavour and a smooth texture as well as giving us a feeling of fullness.

29 Diets high in fat, particularly when combined with a lack of exercise, can cause you to become overweight – a major cause of cancer. But eating too much fat, in itself, might also increase our risk of certain cancers – particularly those of the lung, bowel and prostate – as well as heart disease.

30 As a general rule, saturated fat – found in animal foods like red meat and cheese – is the worst type. Unsaturated fats are the healthier option – these are found in plant foods like vegetables, nuts, seeds and cereals.

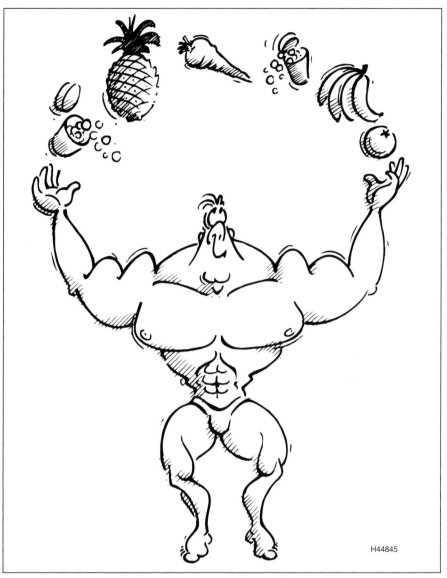

H44845

Fit in 5+ portions of vegetables and fruits each day

2

Easy ways to cut the fat	
Instead of	**Try**
Whole milk	Semi-skimmed or skimmed milk
Biscuits	Dried fruit
Butter	Low fat spread
Fatty meats	Lean meats
Processed meat	Fish or chicken
Chips	Baked potatoes
Cake	Fruit loaf
Ice cream	Frozen yoghurt
Full fat salad dressings	Low fat dressings
Creamy sauces	Tomato-based sauces
Crisps	Home-made popcorn
Tortillas and cream dip	Vegetable crudités with low fat dip
Croissant	Breakfast muffin or crumpet
Mayonnaise	Mustard or chutney

The Mediterranean example

31 Many experts believe that the Mediterranean diet is one of the healthiest around. Not only is it rich in fresh vegetables, fruits and cereals, it also provides some of the best sources of 'good' (unsaturated) fats such as olive and rapeseed oils, avocados, nuts and oily fish. Furthermore, levels of physical activity are often higher in Mediterranean countries.

32 This diet also tends to be low in meat – which can be high in saturated fat. Interestingly, a number of scientific studies have shown that people who regularly eat large portions of red and processed meat have a higher risk of developing cancer, particularly bowel cancer.

33 A good tip to cut down on saturated fats is to begin eating more plant foods – just like our Mediterranean friends – that way, you'll find that you feel full more quickly and have much less room for foods dripping in saturated fats.

Eating out

34 It's easy to blow all your good intentions in a restaurant or when having a take-away. But you should be able to enjoy your food and still choose the healthier options. That way, you'll save the calories, fat and salt and can feel good about yourself at the same time. So what are the healthiest things to order?

Chinese

35 Chinese food can be healthy when meals contain plenty of rice, noodles and vegetables, small meat portions, and tend to have light cooking techniques. Healthy choices:
- Try some of the clear soups with wonton, noodles and vegetables.
- Have steamed rather than fried rice, noodles, dumplings or dim sums.
- Go for dishes with tofu, seafood, poultry or lean meats rather than duck (often served with skin) or pork – both high in fat.

Indian

36 Indian meals can be healthy if they are based on grains, vegetables and fruits, are flavoured with spices and contain small amounts of meat and oil, although many Indian dishes are high in fat. Healthy choices:
- Try meat-free dishes such as dhals (lentil dishes) or saag (spicy spinach).
- Go for yoghurt or tomato-based dishes such as rogan josh or dupiaza.
- Have chapattis, rotis, or naan breads without ghee (clarified butter).
- Tandoori or tikka (dry roasted) chicken is healthy without a creamy sauce.

Italian

37 The Italian diet is typically healthy as it contains plenty of vegetables and fruits, herbs, fish, small amounts of lean meat, pasta, beans, nuts and seeds. Healthy choices:
- Go for tomato-based sauces like napoletana, marinara, pomodoro or arrabiata.
- Try some of the vegetable or seafood soups such as minestrone or Cioppino.
- Use a light sprinkle of Parmesan cheese to add flavour to pasta dishes or pizza.
- Choose thin crust pizza with tomato sauce and vegetable toppings (hold the extra cheese).

Thai

38 Thai meals based on boiled rice, raw or steamed vegetables and fish flavoured with lemon or garlic, are all great choices for healthy eating. Healthy choices:
- Go for low calorie clear soups with noodles, vegetables, lemon grass, herbs or hot and sour soup like tom yum.
- Try spicy Thai salads – often based around seafood and low in fat and calories.
- Order plain boiled rice rather than fried noodles or fried rice, which are high in fat.
- Try dishes with chilli or lemon grass – they add lots of flavour without the fat.

Salt

39 Just like fat, unfortunately the average adult in the UK eats around 8 times the amount of salt his body needs. The tricky part is that over two-thirds of the salt we consume is found in manufactured foods. Things like ready prepared meals, tinned soups, salad dressings, savoury snacks, cooking sauces and stock cubes, as well as canned meat, fish and meat products and many canned vegetables are high in salt which is added during processing. Bread and cereals can also be guilty of containing too much salt. In fact, salt from bread is responsible for almost a quarter of the salt in our diet.

40 We now know that diets high in salt can contribute to high blood pressure and may lead to coronary heart disease,

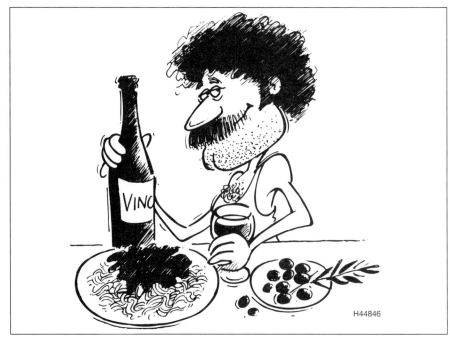

H44846

The Italian diet contains plenty of vegetables and fruits, herbs, fish, small amounts of lean meat, pasta, beans, nuts and seeds

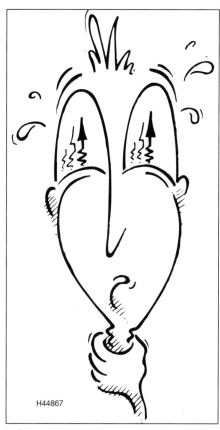

Diets high in salt can contribute to high blood pressure

kidney disease and stroke. Research also shows that salty diets will probably increase our risk of stomach cancer. While we do need some salt for our bodies to function properly, we don't need too much or we could be putting our health at risk.

41 To cut down on adding salt to your food, try hiding the salt cellar and using freshly ground pepper or herbs and spices instead – you'll be surprised how easily you get used to this. Also, try to buy low-salt versions of normally high-salt products like stock-cubes, butter, bacon, baked beans, savoury snacks and soy sauce.

Makes all the difference

42 The average man, consuming around 2,500 calories, should aim to eat less than around 85 grams (3ozs) of total fat a day and no more than 6 grams of salt (sodium). But it's very easy to notch up too much fat and salt without realising it. Here we show how choosing the right shop-bought lunch makes a big difference to the amount of fat and salt you eat.

Original choice	Improved choice
1 wholemeal ham and cheese sandwich	1 wholemeal chicken salad sandwich
1 packet of crisps	1 slice of malt loaf (28g)
1 chocolate mini roll	1 medium apple
1 can of cola	1 glass of pure orange juice (180ml)
Per serving: 870 calories, 38.8 grams fat and 1.42 grams sodium (salt). Contains zero portions of vegetables and fruits.	*Per serving:* 457 calories, 11.3 grams fat and 1.06 grams sodium (salt). Contains 2 portions of vegetables and fruits.

Read the label

43 An easy way to help you keep an eye on the amount of fat and salt you're eating is to know what to look out for on food labels so that you can buy the healthiest choices. Memorise the following and you can impress your friends.

Find it on the label	A Healthy range (per 100g of product)	But watch out for! (per 100g of product)
Total fat	2g – 8g	14g or more
(of which are saturates)	1g – 3g	5g or more
Sodium (salt)	0.1g – 0.3g	0.5g or more

Top 20 superfoods

44 You're probably already asking yourself 'well, what should I buy?'. Although individual foods cannot yet be linked to specific illnesses, we do know that certain foods contain higher than average amounts of nutrients such as vitamin C, selenium, vitamin E and other 'bioactive compounds' – all of which have been shown to help protect against cancer.

45 Here is a list of the 'top 20 superfoods for good health'. Try to include as many of these as you can each time you go food shopping. Bear in mind that this is not a definitive list, and that the foods are not ranked in any particular order. Each food has been chosen because it is believed to help boost the body's immune system, thereby keeping it strong and resistant to serious illnesses such as cancer or heart disease.

- Bean sprouts.
- Brazil nuts.
- Broccoli.
- Brussels sprouts.
- Cabbage.
- Garlic.
- Kiwi fruit.
- Mango.
- Onions.
- Orange peppers.
- Oranges.
- Red peppers.
- Spinach.
- Strawberries.
- Sunflower seeds.
- Sweet potatoes.
- Tomatoes.
- Virgin olive oil.
- Watercress.
- Wholegrain bread.

Lifestyle checks: No smoke without fire

46 Okay, so you've heard it all before. But don't turn the page yet. This advice could add years to your life, never mind helping to improve the way you look, feel and smell.

47 Smoking can lead to all sorts of serious health problems, including heart disease, stroke, various cancers (such as lung, bladder, mouth and throat cancers), bronchitis and emphysema. Our advice is the same as everyone else's. Plain and simple: if you smoke, try to give up. And, if you don't smoke, don't start.

48 On a more positive note, what you may not know is that the very moment you stop smoking, your health will start to improve. After only 20 minutes of not smoking, your blood pressure and pulse return to normal. In just 48 hours, your body is nicotine free and carbon monoxide is cleared from your system. And, within 2 to 12 weeks, your circulation improves and you'll feel noticeably fitter.

49 Best of all, within five years your risk of lung cancer will have dropped

2

dramatically. And your risk may be halved by the time you reach your tenth year of being cigarette-free.

It is believed that smoking causes a third of all cancer deaths.

How much could I save?

50 Because nicotine is highly addictive, many people find it hard to stop smoking. But there are around 12 million ex-smokers in the UK – a living testimony that the habit can be beaten. And these people have since been enjoying the financial – not just physical – benefits of their new tobacco-free lives. If you smoke 20 cigarettes a day, stopping could save you around £1,600 a year. That's a great holiday each year or, over the course of the next five years, a nice new car.

New stress relievers

51 You're more likely to turn to alcohol or cigarettes when you're feeling stressed. But did you know that these fake 'stimulants' can leave you even more stressed? They speed up your heart rate and pulse, and leave you feeling worse afterwards. It makes sense to start thinking of alternative ways of relaxing. Try playing golf or darts with your mates, running, cooking, renting a DVD or going to a footie match – whatever helps you unwind . Or, if you have an open mind, try meditation, acupuncture or yoga – women swear by these. Finding new ways to chill out can make it easier to stop smoking – and may even increase the chances of you never lighting up again. Now wouldn't that be good?

It is estimated that smoking causes as many as 90% of lung cancer cases.

How to give up

- Make a list of the benefits of giving up and look at this regularly to motivate yourself. These might be better all-round health, improved breathing, the chance of living longer, having more money, better skin, or even just smelling better.
- Try to change your way of thinking –

don't think of 'giving up smoking' as that suggests deprivation. Instead, try to think of 'freeing yourself from your addiction'.

- Draw up an action plan by deciding which tactics you'll use to help you succeed. For instance, willpower, nicotine replacement therapy (patches, inhaler or gum), an alternative therapy (such as acupuncture or hypnosis), or a stop smoking clinic (ask your GP for details). Simply choose the method that best suits you and your lifestyle.
- Get professional help – call the NHS Stop Smoking Helpline for advice or Quitline. Alternatively, log onto websites inspired by hundreds of ex-smokers in the UK. See below for details.
- Set a date to stop and commit to it. Then throw out all your ashtrays and lighters and begin to enjoy the nicer aroma in your house.

Scientists estimate that the incidence of mouth, throat, laryngeal (voice-box) and oesophageal (gullet) cancers could be reduced by almost 90% by not smoking, reducing the amount of alcohol you drink and increasing the amount of vegetables and fruits you eat.

Watch your waist

52 Chances are you want to be slimmer – statistics show that the majority of men are overweight. But the important thing is not to aim too high – let's face it, that six-pack is probably long gone. Instead, try to be more realistic and just aim for a healthy weight for your height and size. It's all down to a simple formula: energy in (food) must be balanced by energy out (activity). If there is an excess of either, you'll either gain or lose weight.

53 Most of us probably know that being overweight will increase our risk of heart disease. But did you know that, if you exercised regularly and avoided being overweight, you'd also be helping to reduce your risk of developing cancer? Researchers think they now know why. Being overweight and inactive produces hormonal and metabolic changes that create favourable conditions for cancer to begin. See Section 1 for details.

In the UK, nearly two-thirds of men are currently overweight and one in four is obese – and these numbers are expected to rise over the next decade.

Portion distortion

54 Without realising it, it's easy to overeat. For example, a sensible amount of pasta as a main dish is around 2 cups (cooked volume). But some of us can have as many as four cups without even thinking about it. As for meat, the amount you have on your plate should be no more than 3 oz (which looks like a deck of cards) and as for cheese, 1 oz (which looks like a domino). Again, it's easy to eat twice or three times that amount. But you're doing yourself no favours by stuffing yourself.

55 Also, if it's a habit of yours to have second helpings every time you eat, this is something you should try to become more aware of and change. After a while, you will find you get used to more normal sized portions. And, with this change, you will eat less calories which will lead to weight loss. It'll all be worth it when you begin to see your toes again.

Smart shopping for weight loss

- Believe it or not, what you have in your fridge and cupboards can determine your weight. If they're packed full of unhealthy, high fat foods, then the likelihood is you'll look just like that – fat and unhealthy!
- Turn over a new leaf today by getting rid of the less healthy foods in your cupboards and fridge. You know the culprits – pork pies, Danish pastries, sausage rolls, sweets and biscuits.
- Instead, make sure your fridge and cupboards contain lots of healthy plant foods. This is one of the easiest ways to reduce the number of calories you eat.
- Before you go food shopping, make a detailed list of what you will need for the week. It may help to draw up a menu in advance. Also, make sure you don't go on an empty stomach, as you may be tempted down the chocolates and cakes aisle!
- Make the vegetable and fruit section of the supermarket your first stop. Fill your shopping trolley with a variety

from each of the colour groups: red, orange, yellow, green, purple and white.

- Next, stock up on plenty of grains (go for wholemeal or brown wherever possible) and pulses (such as baked beans and lentils).
- You may then want some low fat animal foods such as semi- or skimmed milk, reduced fat cheese, eggs, fish, poultry and lean meats. But, remember that these foods should only take up a small proportion of your shopping trolley, with the rest filled with plant foods (vegetables, fruits, cereals, grains and beans).
- Last, but not least, don't forget to include some healthy snacks such as low fat yoghurt, rice cakes, vegetable soup, raw vegetables (to chop up and eat on their own, or with a healthy dip), dried fruit and nuts. Have these on hand to nibble on in case you are ever hungry in-between meals – snacking is often where people go wrong when trying to lose weight.

A simple equation

56 Forget fad diets. It's simple: the only way to lose weight – and keep it off – is to eat less and move more. Studies have shown that combining both is the best way to lose weight – and keep it off for good. If you follow the weight loss tips below, you should achieve a healthy weight loss of around 1 lb a week:

a) *Reduce your portion sizes.*
b) *Eat mainly plant foods (vegetables, fruits, cereals, pasta, rice and beans).*
c) *Only eat when you are truly hungry, not just when you're bored, tired or stressed.*
d) *Choose low fat foods (see later on).*
e) *Cut back on the amount of alcohol you drink (see later).*
f) *Exercise every day for at least half an hour, building up to an hour.*

Regular maintenance work

57 Ask anyone who has lost weight, and kept it off. They're more than likely to tell you that their secret is regular exercise. But there's more to exercise than just weight loss. Research now shows strong evidence that people who are regularly active are less likely to develop cancer.
58 As well as preventing the occurrence of cancer, heart disease, stroke, osteoporosis, and being overweight,

regularly moving your body can also help to give you more energy; improve the tone of your muscles; improve the quality of your sleep and help you to relax and deal better with stress. Despite all these benefits, modern life makes it hard to give our bodies the attention they deserve. Two miles is a walkable distance but we now take the car for 50 per cent of such journeys. Also, many jobs are desk-bound and require us to sit still for hours each day.

How much is enough?

59 Whilst all physical exercise is beneficial, to help prevent cancer experts advise that you keep moderately active for at least an hour every day. But you don't have to be a marathon runner. Moderate exercise is relatively easy. It includes things like walking, gentle cycling, even DIY – anything that just gets your heart pumping a little faster. On top of this, you'll need to exercise more energetically for at least one hour each week – most people find the weekend is best for this type of activity. More vigorous exercise includes jogging, swimming or brisk walking.
60 The good news is that you don't have to do your exercise all in one go. As long as you've been active for an hour over the course of the day – plus one hour of more energetic exercise once a week –

your health will improve. And you don't necessarily have to start doing the recommended amount from the word go. Just think of it as a goal to work up to over the next few months. A few simple lifestyle changes, such as leaving the car at home and walking, or taking the stairs instead of the lift, could quickly help you on your way. Before you know it, you'll be feeling better and friends will start noticing how good you look.

The human body is designed to be active. It has over 650 muscles, which contract and relax to make thousands of different movements. From our hearts to our hamstrings, our muscles become stronger and more effective the more we use them.

What counts?

61 For an hour's moderate activity, simply do all the things you usually do, but do them with a little more energy. Put in some extra effort so that your pulse rate increases, you feel slightly warm and breathe a little harder and faster. Brisk walking, walking up stairs, washing the car and digging the garden are all healthy, worthwhile activities.
62 When it comes to your hour's worth

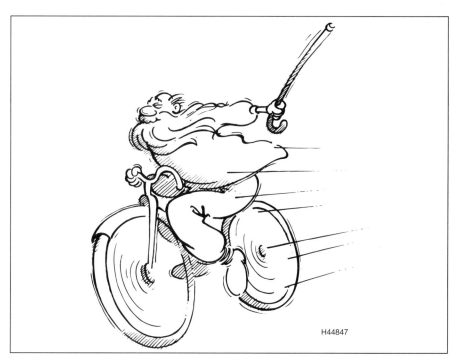

H44847

Look for activities that you enjoy and can fit into your weekly routine

2

of more energetic exercise, look for activities that you enjoy and can fit into your weekly routine. Cycling, swimming, five-a-side football, jogging, tennis or working out in the gym are all excellent choices. The key is to increase your pulse rate enough to make you feel hot and sweaty.

Being physically active throughout life is known to protect against colon cancer and may also protect against lung cancer.

Fitting it in

63 Use lunch times to walk around and clock-up some moderate activity. Getting from A to B is also an easy way to fit in some extra activity. Most people can comfortably walk one mile in 20 minutes – perhaps you could make time to walk to places where you would normally take the car or public transport?
64 If you have a desk job, it's really important to take a lunch-break. An hour's break should give you enough time to complete a third or even half of your 60-minute target for daily moderate or weekly vigorous activity. You can get changed, go for a brisk walk or jog, even fit in a short session in the swimming pool or at the gym, before having a quick shower and getting back to work. You'll feel really great – and smug – by the time you get back to your desk.

I would exercise, if only I wasn't...

Too old

- It's not age that determines physical fitness, it's desire. Whether you're 20, 50 or 90 years old, you can improve your activity levels and enjoy better mobility as well as independence.

Too busy

- Try ten-minute bursts throughout the day to build up your total. It is estimated that three hours of life can be gained for every hour of exercise. And more importantly, quality of life is improved.

Too tired

- Next time you feel tired, go for a walk or a cycle. Providing you aren't unwell, it will leave you feeling invigorated and, at the same time, improve your long-term resistance to colds and illness.

Too unfit

- We all have to start somewhere. No matter how unfit you think you are, you can always improve. You'll be congratulated, as well as respected, for even trying.

Experts agree that a mainly plant-based diet (one that is based around foods that come from plants such as vegetables, fruits, wholegrains and beans), combined with regular physical activity and maintaining a healthy body weight, can reduce the numbers of new cases of cancer by as much as 40 per cent.

More harmful than you think?

65 If you're confused about current drinking advice, it's not surprising. The message is far from straightforward and comes with a number of caveats. The slogan, 'drinking is good for your heart' has become accepted as fact by many people. It's thought that alcohol raises levels of 'good' cholesterol in the blood. This helps prevent arteries clogging, thereby reducing the risk of heart disease.
66 But what most of us don't know is that this benefit is only important for men over 40 or post-menopausal women – in short, those who already have a greater risk of heart disease. Also, only one to two drinks a day are required to provide the protective effects – drinking above this will actually raise blood pressure, thereby increasing the risk of stroke, heart failure and liver disease.
67 When it comes to cancer prevention, it is a more serious matter. In fact, alcohol is classified as a class one carcinogen (cancer-causing substance). That's why cancer experts tell us to drink very little alcohol – or none at all.
68 The bottom line? If you're concerned about preventing cancer, you should ideally not drink alcohol. Despite this, the fact is many of us enjoy a drink when we're out with friends, or at home. If you want to continue drinking, try to limit the amount you have. Although you may find this difficult to begin with, after a few weeks it should get easier – and your liver will thank you for it.

What if you drink too much?

69 Besides feeling rotten on a continual basis, excessive drinking can lead to all sorts of long-term health problems, including;

- *Weight gain:* alcohol is very high in calories and has virtually no

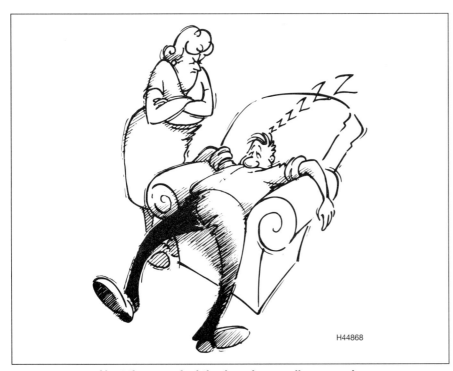

Next time you feel tired, go for a walk or a cycle

nutritional value. Even moderate drinking can lead to weight problems.

- *Liver disease:* the liver is the organ most vulnerable to damage from alcohol because it is responsible for breaking down and eliminating toxins. Heavy drinking can lead to permanent scarring of the liver, commonly known as liver cirrhosis.
- *Cancer:* alcohol is a cancer causing substance. It is known to increase your risk of cancers of the mouth, pharynx, larynx, throat, oesophagus and liver. Alcohol may also increase the risk of bowel cancer. If you drink and smoke, you're putting yourself at an even greater risk.
- *Heart disease:* it is thought that moderate drinking (1-2 drinks a day) may actually help to prevent this disease. However, the benefits tend to apply mostly to men over 40 and post-menopausal women. Also, there is evidence that alcohol makes you more likely to get other diseases of the circulatory system, such as high blood pressure and stroke.

Experts recommend that men should drink no more than two units of alcohol a day.

So what is a drink?

70 A 'drink' counts as one unit of alcohol. The following measures of drink all contain approximately one unit:

- Half a pint of **ordinary** strength lager, beer or cider 3-4% ABV.
- One single pub measure (25ml) spirits 40% ABV.
- One small glass (125ml) wine 8-11% ABV.

Tips to help you drink less

- Keep a drinks diary – this will help you to identify how much you drink and which situations encourage drinking.
- Eat while you drink – better still, eat beforehand as food slows down the rate at which the body absorbs alcohol.
- Dilute your drinks – water down white wine with soda to make a refreshing spritzer; with spirits, increase the amount of mixer you have.

- Don't drink alcohol first – on warm days, have a refreshing non-alcoholic drink to start with, preferably water, to quench thirst – alcohol will only dehydrate you further.
- Pace yourself – make an effort to drink slowly and drink water or a soft drink in between alcoholic drinks.
- Try to have some alcohol-free days during the week.

Still can't cut down?

71 If you are drinking more than you intend and cannot control the urge to drink, call Drinkline for more practical advice. See below for details.

Other things that may surprise you

72 There are just a few other things to be aware of if you want to stay cancer-free for as long as possible. To start with, it's important to be aware of the damage that can be done by overcooking food. Believe it or not, burnt or even charred food – often produced when barbecuing – can contain carcinogens (cancer-causing substances).

73 If you like to have barbecues during the summer, that's fine. Just try not to cook your food directly in the flame.

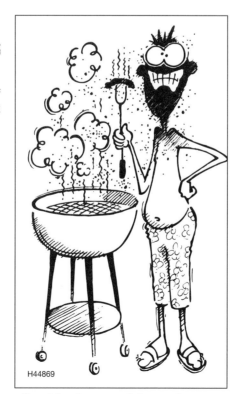

H44869

Burnt food can contain carcinogens (cancer-causing substances)

Wrapping it in foil before cooking, or marinating it before cooking will help to minimise the chances of charring.

74 Try also to avoid eating salt-cured, pickled and smoked foods too often. This may come as a surprise but foods prepared in this way have been shown to increase your risk of cancer.

75 When it comes to pesticides, the golden rule is to wash all your vegetables and fruits thoroughly before eating. Some people think that pesticide residues cause cancer but current research shows that this is unlikely. In the UK, their use is properly regulated and, at present, the levels of additives and residues in our food are not known to affect cancer risk. It is also unlikely that food additives, such as preservatives, colourings or flavourings, significantly affect our cancer risk.

76 Last but not least, sitting in the sun – unprotected – is a major risk factor for skin cancer. Although you probably already knew this, did you also know that it's not just sunbathing in hot climates that can give you cancer? Even in winter and here, in the UK, you can develop skin cancer if you don't take necessary precautions. So cover up, put on some sunscreen when the sun is shining and whatever you do…don't fall asleep in the sun!

Simple checks

77 Today, one of the key health challenges facing men in the UK is cancer. The ironic thing is, although we're more likely than women to die from the disease, we're actually much less likely to go to the GP with symptoms. Is it fear or sheer embarrassment? We just don't know. But we do know that men are generally less well-informed about health issues than women, meaning we're less likely to spot warning signs of system failure.

78 According to a MORI poll, eight out of ten men admitted that they wait too long to ask for medical help. This is recognised as one of the core problems surrounding men's health. The subsequent delay in the reporting of symptoms means that potentially fatal cancers tend to be more advanced in many men when treatment finally begins. The bottom line with cancer prevention: the sooner you act on a symptom and report it to your GP, the better the

2

chances that you will recover. So don't bury your head in the sand or think it'll go away.

79 If you notice something different, be brave and get yourself checked out as soon as you notice any changes. If we were talking about your car, would you ignore it if your fan belt broke, or if the battery went dead? No, you'd be out with the spanners or onto your local garage before it became more serious.

A load of balls

80 Testicular cancer is the most common form of cancer in young men aged 15-45. Although this cancer is still rare, it is affecting more men each year. Fortunately testicular cancer is nearly always curable. And if it is found early on, the treatments needed are very simple – see Chapter 7. If you check your testicles regularly you will get to know how they normally look and feel, and so be able to spot anything unusual.

81 A good time to do this is after a bath or shower when the scrotal skin is relaxed. Most testicular changes prove not to be cancerous or harmful, but even the smallest changes to your testes should be checked by a doctor, just to be on the safe side.

Do it yourself

82 Stand in front of a mirror and assess the size and shape of both testicles. Look carefully. It's common to have one slightly larger, or one that hangs lower.

83 Feel for any changes:

a) *Hold your scrotum in the palm of your hand.*

b) *Place your fingers under the testicle and your thumb on top. You should be able to feel a soft, tender tube at the top and back of the testicle. This is the epididymis that carries and stores sperm.*

c) *Gently roll the testicle between thumb and fingers. It should be smooth, with no lumps or swellings. Compare one testicle with the other, they should both feel the same.*

84 Changes to watch for:

• Any hard lump on a testicle.
• Swelling, enlargement or increase in firmness of a testicle.
• A feeling of heaviness in the scrotum.
• Pain or discomfort in a testicle or the scrotum.
• A dull ache in the groin.
• Any unusual difference between one testicle and the other.

85 If you do find anything unusual, don't be embarrassed, but make an appointment to see your doctor as soon as possible. Your doctor will be able to tell if a change is harmless or more serious. If it is serious, it will need to be treated right away.

Cancer screening tests

86 At the moment, in the UK there is no national screening programme to detect cancers in men. (See the Reference Chapter for the latest situation.) In fact, there is an ongoing debate as to the usefulness of screening, in particular in relation to prostate and bowel cancers. Factors that come into the 'to screen or not to screen' argument include:

• Accuracy of the test (false positive and negative results).
• Evidence that screening saves lives (early detection of cancer does not necessarily mean cure).
• Priority of the costs of screening over, for example, lifestyle prevention and treatments.

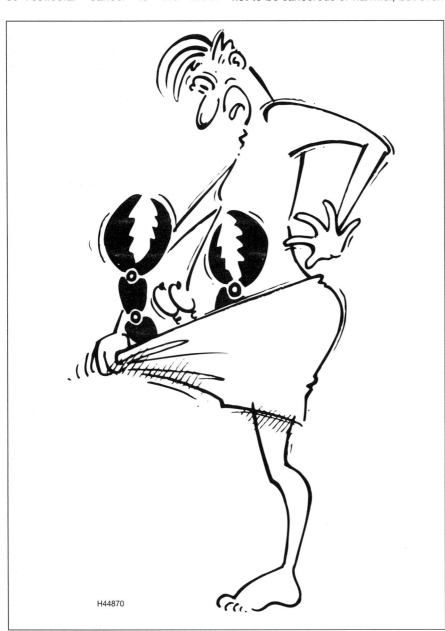

H44870

Testicular cancer is the most common form of cancer in young men aged 15-45

87 It's important to be aware of the early symptoms and to visit your doctor if you are worried, but you will not be routinely screened unless your doctor thinks that you are particularly at risk. This makes it even more important that you – the owner – carry out your own regular bodywork checks to make sure that everything is running smoothly.

PSA blood test

88 Prostate cancer is the commonest cancer among men and affects over 27,000 men each year. It is understandable, then, that some of you might be concerned if the disease has affected a close member of your family, even though you feel fit and healthy and have no symptoms. In these circumstances, a visit to the GP to discuss the options is definitely recommended. Although the GP may choose to give advice and guidance, he or she may suggest a blood test.

89 Used in combination with a digital rectal examination (DRE), the PSA (prostate specific antigen) test is a blood test that checks levels of a protein called PSA, a high level of which can be an indication of prostate cancer; the trouble is that PSA can also be raised in conditions that are not cancerous and so there is a problem of 'false positives'.

90 You may be surprised to learn that a third of men over the age of 50, and nearly all men over the age of 80, have some cancer cells in their prostate gland. Often, these prostate cancers don't need treatment as they are so slow growing that they would not cause any undue problems in a man's lifetime – in fact, the treatment itself could result in side-effects more serious than the disease. For these reasons, the Department of Health is not recommending a national screening programme using PSA tests.

Screening for bowel cancer

91 Again, in the UK national screening programmes are not currently recommended for this cancer. Effective early detection of bowel cancer would involve regular colonoscopy (a bendy telescope examination), which is a costly procedure. So far, no-one has come up with a good enough reason to spend this money, as current research does not suggest that many lives would be saved.

92 A much more basic screening test is a faecal occult blood test. This involves using a simple kit to detect blood that is not visible to the naked eye in the faeces. The effectiveness of these, though, is in dispute as 'false positives' and 'false negatives' (due to tumours bleeding only intermittently) are possible and a positive result could arise for many reasons, not just cancer.

93 In people who have a high risk of bowel cancer, screening can be appropriate. If you have a close relative (sibling, parent or child) who developed bowel cancer before the age of 45, then you have a one in ten lifetime risk of developing the condition yourself. If you have two or more close relatives with this type of cancer then the risk increases to one in six. For these people, regular colonoscopy is usually recommended.

General symptoms to watch for

94 If you are a smoker, it's also a good idea to regularly check your mouth – including your gums and tongue – for any unusual sores, growths, swellings or white patches.

95 Smoker or not, you should check your skin for the development of any moles (new ones or changes to existing ones). Don't forget your lower legs, the soles of the feet or the back, as these are areas that we don't often look at. Perhaps get a partner or friend to do this for you.

96 If you are at all concerned by any change in your body, visit your GP as soon as possible. The earlier cancer is detected, the more successful the treatment may be.

97 Many symptoms that might indicate cancer are also just as likely to be caused by a less serious illness. But it's always better to be safe. If you experience any of the following for more than a couple of weeks, you should visit your GP:
- A noticeable, persistent change in bowel or bladder habits, for no apparent reason.
- A sore or bruise that does not heal as normal.
- Unusual bleeding or discharge from your bottom.
- A thickening or lump in the breast, testicle, or anywhere else in the body.
- Persistent indigestion or difficulty in swallowing.

- A significant change – in size, texture or colour – of a wart or mole.
- A persistent nagging cough or hoarseness.
- Coughing up blood.
- Vomiting.
- Significant weight loss (for no apparent reason).

Keeping on track

98 Okay, so you've won the battle of the bulge, conquered the evil weed and people are beginning to comment about that halo round your head. It sounds like congratulations are in order. Make sure you treat yourself to a holiday or some new kit as a slap on the back. This is the ideal scenario. For most of you, however, it's probably a long path to a healthier lifestyle – and you may have had lots of relapses along the way. Don't be too disheartened. It takes time to change long-established habits so give yourself a break.

99 What you need to do now is learn more about your unhealthy habits. Think about which aspects you find particularly difficult to change and start taking these into account in the future. Perhaps you're being too hard on yourself and unrealistic? Sometimes long-term change means breaking your goals into chunks, rather than chewing off a big bite at one go.

Set new action lists

100 The important thing is to keep challenging yourself so that you stay motivated. Your targets should push you a little harder each time. But it's also important that you enjoy your new lifestyle. Try to keep up your interest by regularly trying new varieties of healthy foods. And pep up your exercise routine by trying a new sport, or buying yourself some new exercise clothes. Think about what you've gained – a better body, new friends, better health. Think of all the benefits that you have been enjoying as a result of switching to a healthier diet and lifestyle.

Dealing with lapses

101 Ever ordered a greasy takeaway when you're trying to lose weight? Or drunk way too much, when you've been making an effort to cut down? Most of us have done this, or something similar. Again, don't be too hard on yourself. Lapses are an inevitable part of life –

2

particularly when you're trying to change a habit of a lifetime. Just make a concerted effort not to allow these 'slips' to throw you. The important thing is that they don't lead to a complete relapse to your old habits.

102 And don't be too strict on yourself. For instance, once you get your weight down, you should be able to have a takeaway every now and then. The odd takeaway can still have a place in an otherwise healthy eating pattern. The crucial thing is to avoid feeling deprived – this can sometimes lead to a relapse.

Further information

103 If you would like to know more, look at the contacts section at the back of this book, or contact:

NHS Stop Smoking Helpline
0800 169 0 169

Quitline
0800 002 200

Websites inspired by hundreds of ex-smokers in the UK
www.ash.org.uk
www.sickofsmoking.com

Drinkline
0800 917 8282

NHS Giving Up Smoking web site
www.givingupsmoking.co.uk

Chapter 3
Air intake system (respiratory)

Contents

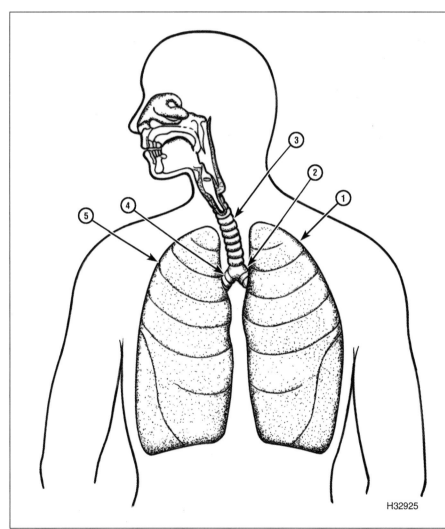

The lungs and bronchi

1 Left lung   2 Left bronchus   3 Trachea   4 Right bronchus   5 Right lung

1 Lung Cancer

Introduction

1 Most people think of the lungs as two plastic bags or balloons. Nothing could be further from the truth. Lungs are complex structures with more similarity to sponges than balloons. The main pipe (bronchus) connects both lungs to the airway in the throat. It splits lower in the chest, branching increasingly until tiny blind-ending pockets are reached. These are the alveoli where oxygen is exchanged for carbon dioxide across the thin membranes. Cancer can arise in the fine tubes but mainly in the larger tubes, the bronchi.

2 The correct medical term for lung cancer is bronchial carcinoma, a cancer of the large tubes of the lung. The lining cells of the air tubes in healthy lungs are tall (columnar) and the surfaces nearest the inside of the tube are covered with fine hairs (cilia) which move together. Imagine a wind blowing across a field of ripe corn. The movement of the cilia acts to carry dust, smoke particles and other foreign material upwards and away from the deeper parts of the lungs. This is essential to keep the lungs clear of debris and potentially harmful particles.

3 Smoking cigarettes damages the ability of the lining cells to do their jobs. First, the cilia disappear, then the number of cells increases, and finally the

3

cells become flattened, so that the columnar lining is replaced by an abnormal scaly layer. Some years later this layer may develop into bronchial carcinoma.

4 Lung cancer is uncommon before the age of 40. Only about 1 case in 100 is diagnosed in people younger than 40. The great majority of cases (85 per cent) occur in people over 60.

5 The outlook in lung cancer is not good. After diagnosis of the disease only 20 per cent are alive a year later, and only 8 per cent, overall, survive for five years.

Symptoms

6 Lung cancer usually shows itself with a productive cough, often with a little blood in the sputum. There may also be breathlessness. Pain in the chest is common, especially if the cancer has spread to the lung lining (pleura) or the chest wall.

7 Unfortunately the tumour may show no signs until late in its development. Watch out for:
- A persistent cough.
- Coughing up blood-stained phlegm (sputum).
- Shortness of breath.
- Chest discomfort.
- Repeated bouts of pneumonia or bronchitis.
- Loss of appetite.
- Loss of weight.

8 These don't necessarily mean you have cancer, but they need your doctor's attention in case you need further tests.

Causes

9 It is almost entirely due to cigarette smoking, either directly or through passive smoking. The rate of lung cancer in non-smokers rises significantly if they are regularly exposed to other people's cigarette smoke.

Diagnosis

10 Unfortunately diagnosis tends to be late in the day and can be fairly obvious from the symptoms you describe to your doctor. X-ray examination will often confirm the diagnosis, although sometimes it is also necessary to examine the inside of the bronchi with an instrument called a bronchoscope. If a tumour is seen, a sample (biopsy) is usually taken for examination to see what type it is. Cancer cells can sometimes be found in the sputum.

Treatment

11 Treatment will depend on the type of cancer, how developed it is and your general state of health. Surgery, radiotherapy and chemotherapy may be used alone or together to treat cancer of the lung.
- Surgery: removal of part or all of the lung.
- Radiotherapy: the use of radiation treatment to destroy cancer cells.
- Chemotherapy: the use of drugs that kill cancer cells.

12 Nobody is trying to kid you that any of these treatments guarantee a cure, but early detection of the cancer can make all the difference.

13 Better still, reduce your risks of getting lung cancer in the first place by stopping smoking.

First the good news: Lung cancer in men, caused almost entirely by smoking, is preventable and on the decrease.
Now the bad news: Young men think they are immune.

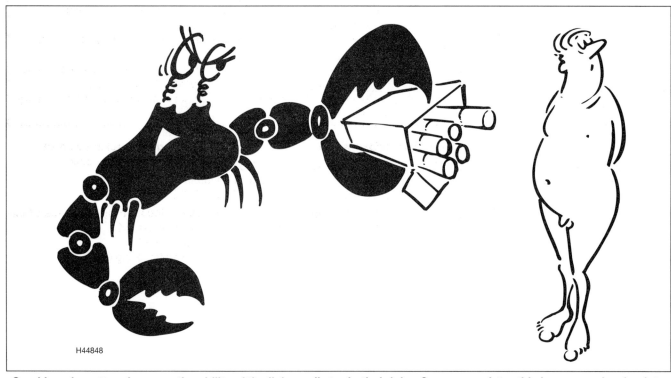

H44848

Smoking cigarettes damages the ability of the lining cells to do their jobs. Some years later this layer may develop into bronchial carcinoma

Around 80,000 people develop lung cancer in the UK each year and most of them are men. Yet of all the cancers it has to be one of the most preventable.

The Smoking Gun

14 It's not difficult to work out what causes it. If you don't smoke, your chances of getting lung cancer are very small. Start early, die early and the amount of tobacco you smoke also shifts you that bit closer to the great scrapyard in the sky.

15 Filters and low tar protect you? Aye, and sugar-coated cyanide won't kill you either. Wise up and stub it out.

So go for pipes and cigars? No way, they just give you a feeling of false security. Cut down then? No, that doesn't work either. You gradually creep back up. Stop completely.

16 All over the UK men are getting the message. That's why lung cancer in men is on the decrease. You can be one of them.

You do not get permanently fat when you stop but you do enjoy your food more.

How to quit the weed

- Nicotine patches and other ways of helping you to stop can be obtained through your GP. These can be very successful in easing the craving for nicotine.
- Get in touch with self-help groups or organisations which supply information.
- If you can't do it for yourself, do it for your partner or kids.

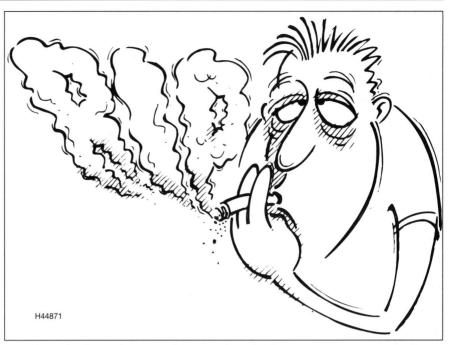

H44871

If you don't smoke, your chances of getting lung cancer are very small

Quit plan

- Set a day and date to stop. Tell all your friends and relatives, they will support you.
- Like deep sea diving, always take a buddy. Get someone to give up with you. You will reinforce each other's will power.
- Clear the house and your pockets of any packets, papers or matches.
- One day at a time is better than leaving it open-ended.
- Map out your progress on a chart or calendar. Keep the money saved in a separate container.
- Chew on a carrot. Not only will it help you do something with your mouth and hands, it provides a great chat up line for women. 'What's up Doc?'
- Ask your friends not to smoke around you. People accept this far more readily than they used to do.

Further information

17 If you would like to know more, look at the contacts section at the back of this book, or contact:

NHS Stop Smoking Helpline
An advisor can put you in touch with your local NHS Stop Smoking Service.
0800 169 0 169

NHS Giving Up Smoking web site
www.givingupsmoking.co.uk

Quitline
0800 002 200

Websites inspired by hundreds of ex-smokers in the UK
www.ash.org.uk
www.sickofsmoking.com

3

Notes

Chapter 4
Hydraulic system (blood)

Contents

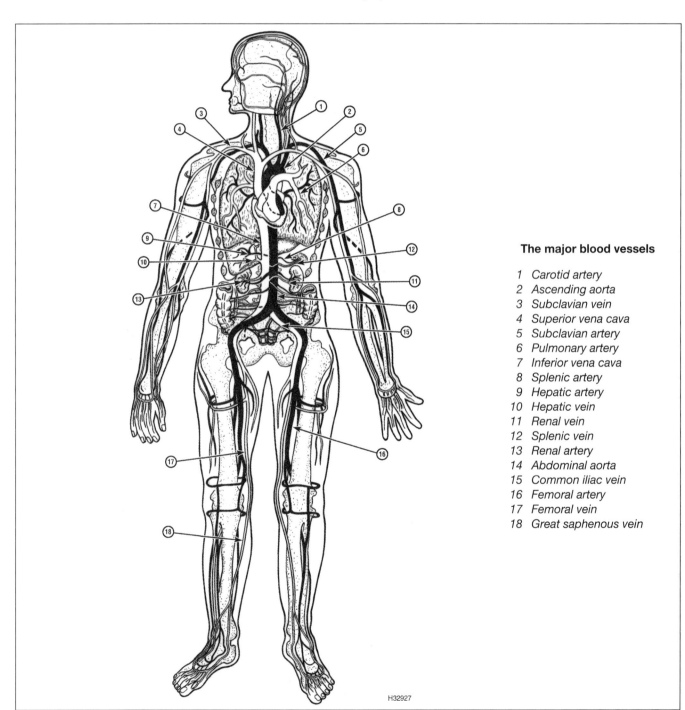

The major blood vessels

1 Carotid artery
2 Ascending aorta
3 Subclavian vein
4 Superior vena cava
5 Subclavian artery
6 Pulmonary artery
7 Inferior vena cava
8 Splenic artery
9 Hepatic artery
10 Hepatic vein
11 Renal vein
12 Splenic vein
13 Renal artery
14 Abdominal aorta
15 Common iliac vein
16 Femoral artery
17 Femoral vein
18 Great saphenous vein

H32927

4

1 Leukaemia

Introduction

1 Despite the fear which surrounds this particular cancer, leukaemia is now more treatable than most cancers affecting men, especially when caught early.

2 Blood is made up of basically two types of blood cells – red and white – although this is very simplistic as the white blood cells are actually a complex group of different types of blood cells. Blood is made up in the main by red blood cells, but cancer involves almost exclusively the white blood cells and the term leukaemia comes from two Greek words meaning 'white blood'.

3 The number of different white cell types is reflected by the types of leukaemia. Leukaemia is not one disease, but a group of different diseases. What they have in common is an abnormal production of white blood cells. Blood cells are produced in the marrow of many bones. Leukaemia is a disorder of the blood-forming cells in which certain groups of white blood cells reproduce in the bone marrow in a disorganised and uncontrolled way.

4 Perhaps the most serious effect of this uncontrolled growth is the progressive displacement, and interference with, the normal constituents of the blood. This can have serious implications for normal bone marrow constituents that are crowded out, such as those concerned with red blood cell production, blood clotting and producing the cells of the immune system that protect against infection.

5 What tends to emerge is a complex picture and leukaemia is not the same, therefore, in every person. They are all serious conditions – some more so than others – which, unless effectively treated, can cause anaemia from a shortage of red blood cells, severe bleeding from interference with blood clotting elements such as platelets, or infection from the loss of normal immune

system cells. They also respond differently to treatment, with real cures possible in many cases.

6 There are two main groups:

Acute leukaemias

- Which are in general the more dangerous.

Chronic leukaemias

- In which the outlook is usually much better.

7 Leukaemias can also be split into two large categories depending on their origin:

Acute lymphoblastic (lymphocytic) leukaemias

- Predominantly affecting young children.

Acute myelogenous (myeloid) leukaemias

- Mainly affecting adults. These arise in the bone marrow itself.

Symptoms

8 There are important differences in the way the two basic types of leukaemias – acute and chronic – make themselves felt.

Acute leukaemias

9 As the name suggests, they start suddenly and the man will generally become ill in a matter of days. Symptoms vary but they include:

- Pallor.
- Fever.
- Various infections.
- Influenza-like symptoms, a feeling of great tiredness, sore throat.
- Bleeding from the gums and into the skin with unexplained bruising.
- Loss of appetite and weight.
- Lumps in the neck, armpits and groin caused by the lymph nodes becoming larger.

10 Blood checks may show a severe anaemia, with a significant lack of red blood cells and usually large numbers of white cells in early stages of development. Recognising these cells by microscopy is vital as it will help to decide the best course of treatment.

Chronic leukaemias

11 A slow, insidious onset with gradually developing lassitude and fatigue set these leukaemias apart from the acute forms. Increasing size of the spleen can cause a dragging feeling with pain in the upper left side of the abdomen. There is slow loss of weight, aching in the bones

and possibly nose bleeds or blood in the urine. Some men find warm rooms hard to bear and may sweat heavily, especially at night.

Causes

12 Generally, no specific single cause is known. It seems likely that, in most cases, a number of different factors combine, or interact, to cause the disease. These factors include genetics, radiation, environmental chemicals, and cancer-causing viruses.

13 On the other hand, the cause of some leukaemias is understood. All leukaemic cells in people with chronic myeloid leukaemia, for instance, contain an abnormal chromosome called the Philadelphia chromosome. This is derived from a broken-off piece of chromosome 9 attaching itself to a broken chromosome 22. The result is a gene which generates a protein that disrupts stem cell function in the bone marrow.

14 The association between leukaemia and radiation is well recognised. There is an increased incidence in people who have had a large single dose of radiation, not least those involved in war-time radiation, and in those who have had repeated smaller doses (as in medical treatment). The size of the risk is directly proportional to the total dose of radiation. Even so, even a large dose of radiation does not necessarily cause leukaemia – it only increases the risk. The name of the game is to avoid radiation or expose yourself to it as little as possible.

15 Chemicals such as benzene can damage bone marrow function. This damage is followed by leukaemia.

16 Sadly, treatment with some anti-cancer drugs can also increase the risk of developing leukaemia.

Diagnosis

17 A great deal depends on your symptoms and your doctor's examination. A full examination of your blood sample, and often of a sample of bone marrow too, will be made. The microscopic appearance of the white cells, together with a chromosomal analysis of the abnormal blood cells, will help establish the diagnosis.

Treatment

18 Chemotherapy is still the mainstay and saves thousands of lives. It is especially effective in chronic leukaemias and often maintains life for many years. Removal of the spleen is often advised in chronic leukaemias.

19 Good news for people with acute leukaemias as well. Around 50 to 60 per cent of patients enjoy a remission on chemotherapy. Tackling the anaemia, bleeding tendency and infections which can complicate the condition is essential, and this will usually involve blood transfusions and antibiotics. Other treatments include bone marrow transplants, radiotherapy and white cell transfusions.

20 Undoubtedly the biggest leap forward has come from bone marrow transplants, which are increasingly used to treat leukaemia. The graft provides the person with cancer a fresh supply of stem cells acting as the source of a continuing supply of healthy new red and white blood cells.

21 The donated marrow is obtained from a matched donor such as a sibling. First the abnormal bone is destroyed using total body radiation in combination with the drug cyclophosphamide. Then marrow is sucked out of the marrow cavity of the pelvis or breastbone of the donor and injected into one of the recipient's veins. The marrow cells are carried by the bloodstream to the recipient's bone marrow, where they settle and begin to produce new cell lines (clones) by normal reproduction.

22 In certain forms of leukaemia it is even possible to take marrow from a person in remission, store it, expose the person to heavy radiation and then replace the original sample to start up the marrow function again.

2 Lymphoma

Introduction

1 Lymphoid tissue has a number of roles in the body, not least to attack infections. Most of this takes place in the lymph nodes ('lymph glands') and the spleen. White blood cells, 'lymphocytes', are the most important part of the immune defence system.

2 Once it was thought that all white blood cells were the same, but now we know there are two broad classes of lymphocytes, T cells and B cells, which produce antibodies to attack bacteria and viruses. Lymphomas are cancerous lymphocytes, mainly B cells.

3 There are two kinds of lymphoma: Hodgkin's lymphoma (also called Hodgkin's disease) and non-Hodgkin's lymphoma, which used to be called lymphosarcoma. The lymphatic tissue in Hodgkin's lymphoma contains specific cells – Reed-Sternberg cells – that are not found in any other cancerous lymphomas or cancers. These cells distinguish Hodgkin's from non-Hodgkin's lymphomas. Non-Hodgkin's lymphoma usually consists of identical B lymphocytes which may have come from one single abnormal cell. It can affect any part of the body's lymphatic system, but varies in the speed at which it grows and spreads.

Symptoms

4 One of the problems with Hodgkin's lymphoma is the lack of early signs or symptoms. Enlarged lymph nodes in various places around the body such as in the neck or armpits give some warning and should not be ignored. Weakness, tiredness and a reduced ability to fight off infection tend to come on later in the course of the condition. Younger men tend to develop the cancer most, but the good news is that it is very treatable, especially with early diagnosis.

5 Non-Hodgkin's lymphoma tends to have widespread, painless, firm enlargement of lymph nodes with lumps under the armpits, neck, abdomen or groin. There is also tiredness, loss of weight, and sometimes fever with night-time sweats. These enlarged nodes may put pressure on various structures of the body. This may cause various effects, which include:

- Pressure on the spinal cord with difficulty in moving or pain.
- Swallowing problems.
- Breathing difficulty.
- Vomiting from blockages in the bowel.
- Swelling of limbs from too much fluid.

Cause

6 Lymphomas do not seem to have any direct cause. There appears to be a genetic factor, as it can be more common in some families.

Diagnosis

7 Although the symptoms tend to be vague, the diagnosis is partly made on the clinical signs and symptoms. It may be confirmed by one or more of the following:

- Blood tests, especially checking out the types of cells present.
- Chest X-ray.
- CT scan (computer assisted X-ray examination).
- MRI scan (magnetic resonance imaging which does not use X-rays and can better visualise more detail of the body).
- Microscopic appearance of tissue from a lymph node biopsy – a small sample of tissue taken either by using a fine needle or during surgery.

Prevention

8 Unfortunately we don't know enough about lymphomas to give good advice on prevention, other than avoiding the obvious agents that can cause cancer. Much more important therefore is early diagnosis and seeing your doctor.

Treatment

9 This will depend very much on how early the cancer is diagnosed. When treatment is required, radiotherapy is often best as in many cases this alone is enough.

10 In more severe cases other forms of treatment must be added. Chemotherapy with various combinations of drugs may be given every four weeks for six months. The results are often excellent, but the earlier the diagnosis is made, the better.

4

Chapter 5
Engine management system (brain)

Contents

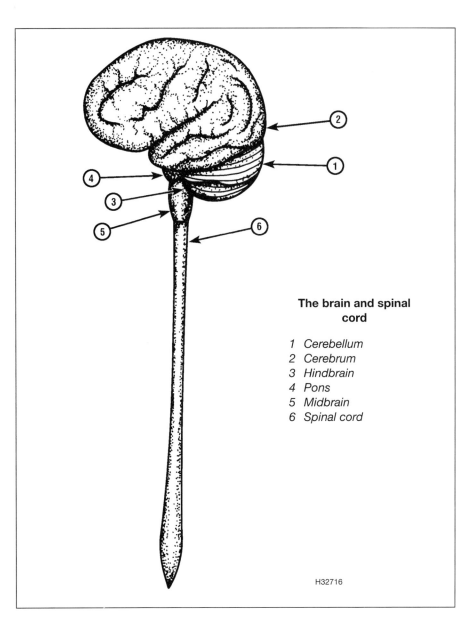

The brain and spinal cord

1 *Cerebellum*
2 *Cerebrum*
3 *Hindbrain*
4 *Pons*
5 *Midbrain*
6 *Spinal cord*

H32716

1 Brain cancer

1 The brain is more than just a huge number of nerve cells. It has a complex support structure of blood vessels and coverings, not to mention bone, which forms an intricate scaffolding within the skull.

2 For reasons not entirely known, nerve cells of the brain do not form cancers. Cancers arise in the structures supporting the brain such as:
• Brain coverings, the meninges (meningioma).
• Neurological supportive tissue, the glial cells (glioma).
• Blood vessels (haemangioma).
• Bone of the skull (osteoma).
• Pituitary gland (pituitary adenoma).

3 By far the most common kind of brain cancers are those spreading to the brain from another malignant tumour in some other part of the body such as the lung, breast or prostate gland.

4 More rare forms of brain cancers are of congenital origin (craniopharyngioma, teratoma) and are due to abnormal development while in the womb.

Symptoms

5 Unlike some other kinds of tumours, the signs and symptoms of a growing tumour within the skull are often indirect and not always obvious until a fairly late stage. A progressive rise in the internal pressure within the skull, either from the growing mass or from interference with

5

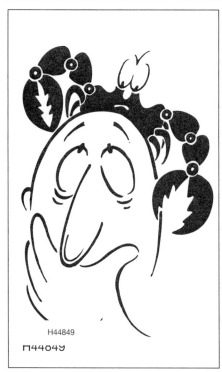

H44849

For reasons not entirely known, nerve cells of the brain do not form cancers

the normal circulation of the cerebrospinal fluid, can put pressure on parts of the brain or its blood supply. This can produce symptoms such as:
* Severe, persistent headaches resistant to even powerful pain killers.
* Persistent dizziness.
* Vomiting which is sometimes sudden, unexpected and often without any feeling of 'sickness' (nausea).
* Seizures (fits), either major seizures or local twitching. Any seizure in a person previously free from them must be checked out by a doctor.
* Loss of part of the field of vision. This can mean poor vision to the side, central loss where you need to look slightly to one side to see properly or loss of vision in one eye.
* Hallucinations, particularly of strange tastes or noises.
* Drowsiness, especially with no good reason and with difficulty to rouse. This can happen in the middle of the day.

* Personality changes or abnormal and uncharacteristic behaviour such as sudden irrational anger or weeping. Emotional 'flatness' where there is a lack of response to other people can also be a symptom.

6 Even so, if every person who had a headache was suffering from a brain tumour there would be standing room only in the hospital neurology units. Headache may be a symptom but only a tiny proportion of even severe headaches are due to brain tumour. A new, persistent and severe headache without any obvious cause can be a different kettle of fish, and in that case you should seek medical attention.

Causes

7 Like many cancers brain tumours can often be very preventable. Cancer from the lung can spread to the brain at an unfortunately early stage in the condition. Lung cancer, and therefore secondary cancer to the brain, is preventable by simply stopping smoking.

8 Cancers arising within the brain itself are thankfully less common but the causes are unknown. Although radiation from mobile phones has attracted much attention, any link with primary brain tumours is not yet confirmed. Banning their use while driving may make more sense than simply preventing accidents, as reducing your exposure to any intense radiation from whatever source must be a good idea.

Diagnosis

9 Most of the diagnosis comes from the symptoms and signs. As the skull is pretty tough and inflexible, any growth inside tends to raise the pressure inside the skull and can cause high blood pressure as the heart tries to force blood into the skull against this back pressure. Checking the retina at the back of the eyes using an ophthalmoscope (a flat telescope) is vital as it is in direct connection with the brain and the only visible way of checking from outside. In one quarter of cases of brain tumour and in most of those with raised pressure within the head, the parts of the optic nerves visible within the retina are obviously swollen (papilloedema).

10 Most people will also be checked by special X-ray or other non-invasive tests such as CT or MRI scanning.

Treatment

11 Once considered virtually impossible, many tumours can now be successfully treated, especially the non malignant variety. The outcome depends on the location, type and degree of malignancy of the tumour. Many brain tumours are not malignant. Treatment is by surgical removal, often supplemented by radiotherapy.

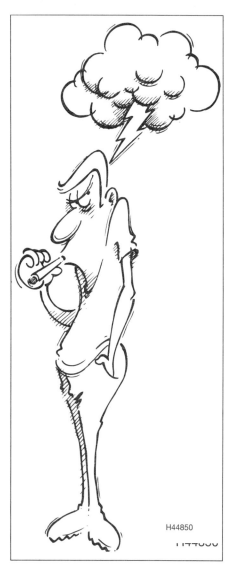

H44850

Lung cancer, and secondary cancer to the brain, is preventable by simply stopping smoking

Chapter 6
Fuel and exhaust (digestive system)

Contents

1 Bowel cancer

This section has been developed by the national charity Beating Bowel Cancer and supported by Merck Pharmaceuticals.

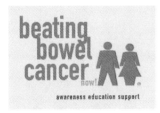

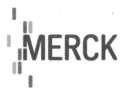

Breaking down taboos

1 To take a stereotype, the British man is well known for his reluctance to talk openly – let alone seek advice – about his own health. With so-called 'embarrassing' problems, the British stiff upper lip is even more tightly pursed. While toilet humour is an accepted form of banter in the office or over a drink, talking about any personal problems related to bottoms is a real no-no for many men – even with health professionals, close family or friends. Language is often a barrier for men trying to describe their symptoms, with words such as 'rectum' or 'diarrhoea' causing acute social embarrassment.

2 Although many people find it embarrassing to talk about symptoms of bowel problems, it is surprising how common they really are. There are lots of common conditions that could cause changes in the workings of the bowels, pain and bleeding from the bottom. In most cases, it won't be cancer.

Don't die of embarrassment – visit your GP without delay if you've been experiencing symptoms for a period of around six weeks

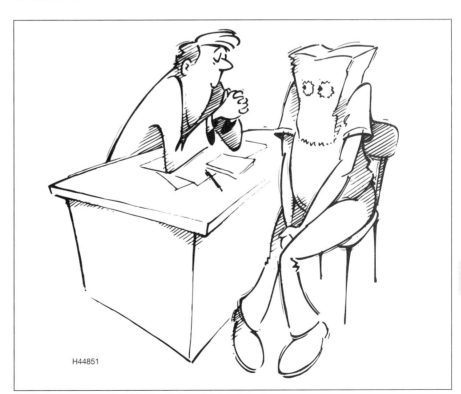

British man is well known for his reluctance to talk openly

6

The scale of the problem

3 Bowel cancer is the second most deadly cancer in the UK – only lung cancer kills more people. Around 35,600 people are diagnosed with the disease each year and over 45% will die as a result. That means that it claims the lives of over 16,000 men and women in the UK each year.

4 However, bowel cancer is one of the most curable cancers if caught early enough. It is estimated that around 80% of cases could be treated successfully if caught at an early stage.

5 Many people, often embarrassed to discuss their symptoms, delay seeking medical advice. It is vital to look out for possible symptoms and have them investigated (by a health professional such as your GP) if they persist.

What is bowel cancer?

6 The large bowel is a question-mark-shaped tube of muscle – about four feet long – which runs from the appendix, via the colon, to the rectum. Bowel cancer is cancer of any part of this tube. If it is not treated, it will increase in size and may cause a blockage, or it can ulcerate, leading to blood loss and anaemia. (The terms 'small bowel' and 'large bowel' reflect the width of the gut rather than its length. For some reason the small bowel is almost immune to cancer compared to the large bowel and rectum, the very last part of the digestive system.)

7 Most cancers start with wart-like growths known as polyps on the wall of the gut. Polyps are very common as we get older – one in ten people over 60 have them. However, most polyps do not turn into cancer. If potentially cancerous polyps can be found at an early stage, they can be removed painlessly without the need for a major operation.

Bowel cancer is more common in men than women, and more men will die from it as well. Part of the reason is later diagnosis.

Don't sit on your symptoms

8 The most common symptoms are change of bowel habit and rectal bleeding. However, these are also common in people who don't have cancer. The facts show that:

*   Nearly 20% of us experience bleeding from the bottom each year.
*   Over a third of us experience

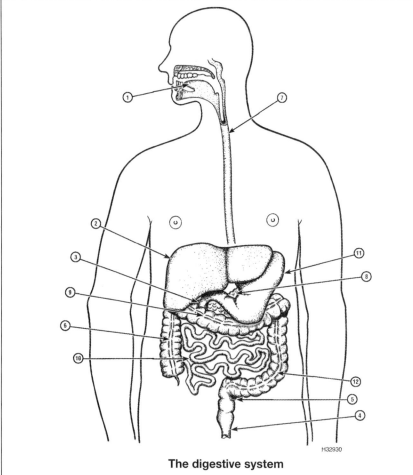

The digestive system

1	Tongue	5	Caecum
2	Liver	6	Ascending colon
3	Duodenum	7	Oesophagus
4	Rectum	8	Pancreas
		9	Transverse colon
		10	Small intestine
		11	Stomach
		12	Descending colon

H32930

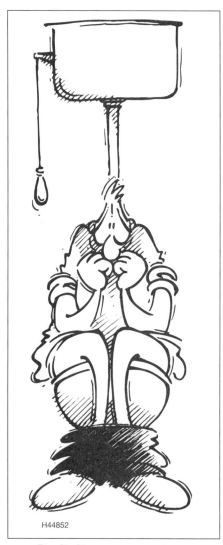

H44852

Don't sit on your symptoms

constipation or diarrhoea at some point in our lives.

Early detection gives the best protection, so know your bum, chum.

Higher risk symptoms – 'watch and wait'

9 If you have any of the higher risk symptoms outlined below, it is safe to 'watch and wait' for up to six weeks. But if they persist, you should get advice from your GP and ask about the possibility of further investigation.

- Change of bowel habit (especially important if you also have bleeding) – a recent, persistent change of bowel habit to looser, more diarrhoea-like motions, going to the toilet or trying to 'go' more often.
- Rectal bleeding – look out for rectal bleeding that persists with no reason. For example, bleeding can be due to piles – but if so you will have other symptoms such as straining with hard stools, a sore bottom, lumps and itching. If you are over 60 piles could be hiding more serious symptoms, so it is especially important to get this investigated.

Other high risk symptoms and signs

- Unexplained anaemia, found by your GP.
- A lump or mass in your abdomen, felt by your GP.
- Persistent, severe abdominal pain which has come on recently for the first time (especially in older people)

What's wrong with me?

10 Most people with these symptoms do not have bowel cancer, but if they persist beyond the 6 week 'watch and wait' period it is very important to have further tests to rule it out.

11 Your symptoms could be caused by the following:

- Piles or haemorrhoids: soft swellings, a bit like spongy varicose veins, which usually have other symptoms such as pain and itching. Bright red bleeding found on the toilet paper or sudden large amounts of blood are almost always caused by piles. Your GP or pharmacist will be able to

recommend a fast and effective over-the-counter treatment
- Polyps: wart-like growths on the bowel lining, which can sometimes cause bleeding. These can be removed painlessly without the need for an operation.
- Fissures: a split or tear in the lining of the gut, sometimes caused by constipation. Fissures can be treated with creams available from the pharmacist
- Crohn's disease: Painful inflammation of the gut, which can put you more at risk of bowel cancer. If you suffer from the condition, you should ask your GP to be monitored regularly for bowel cancer.
- Ulcerative colitis: inflammation of the bowel which can cause bleeding and mucus. This condition can put you at a greater risk from bowel cancer and you should talk to your GP about being monitored.

In the league table of commonest male cancers, bowel cancer comes in at third place after cancer of skin and prostate.

Family history

12 If you ask around in your family, you may well find someone who has had bowel cancer. While bowel cancer can in some cases be put down to genetics, family history doesn't necessarily mean that you are going to get it. In general, the closer the relatives are to you (eg, brother, sister, mother, father, child) and the younger they were diagnosed, the more you need to get it checked out. The following is a guide to the action you may need to take depending on your family history:

One close relative under 45 affected.
- Talk to your GP about screening in your area. It is usually recommended 10 years before the age at which your relative developed the disease.

Two or more close relatives from the same side of the family.
- The younger those relatives, the more need there is for you to discuss screening with your GP.

Less strong family history (such as a grandparent who died in their 70s).
- You are probably not at an increased

risk. However, do talk to your GP if you are worried.

13 Screening for bowel cancer can help to detect polyps, which may be cancerous, at an early stage, and is usually carried out using a simple procedure called a colonoscopy. Alternatively, if you have been diagnosed with cancer, or you have a relative with bowel cancer who is willing to be tested, you might be offered genetic testing if your doctor thinks that your family is likely to have a genetic mutation in one of the known bowel cancer genes.

Your risk increases if there is bowel cancer in the family, but diet and smoking are among the main culprits.

Diet and lifestyle

14 In many cases bowel cancer occurs without any obvious cause. However, experts also suggest that a diet high in red meat and low in fibre, fruit and vegetables can increase the risk of bowel cancer. Obesity, high alcohol consumption and lack of physical exercise may also put you at risk.

Eating healthily

15 A high fibre diet is particularly recognised for reducing the risk of constipation, irritable bowel syndrome and bowel cancer. Fibre is indigestible plant material such as cellulose, lignin and pectin which is found in fruits, vegetables, grains and beans. There are two types of fibre – soluble and insoluble. Fibre provides bulk to your food, helps it pass easily through the gut and also retains water (so making us feel full and therefore we eat less).

16 Reports suggest that we should be eating 18g of fibre each day – yet most of us probably eat much less (around 10-12g). To give a couple of examples, a banana contains 1.8g, as does 1 slice of wholemeal toast.

17 When increasing your fibre intake, start slowly and build up to the recommended level. Here are some tips:

- Replace lower fibre foods with high fibre foods (see chart below), eg, choose whole grain breads and cereals.
- Eat vegetables and fruit raw whenever possible.

6

- Steam or stir-fry vegetables if you need to cook them – boiling can cause up to one half of the fibre to be lost in the water.
- Replace fruit or vegetable juice with the whole fruit – fruit skin and membranes are a particularly good source of fibre.
- Start your day with a bowl of high-fibre cereal (5g of fibre or more per serving). Add fresh fruit or sprinkle with wheat germ or bran for an easy way to build up fibre intake.
- Eat only whole grain products.

Exercise for life

18 Recent research has found compelling evidence that regular exercise could cut the risk of developing bowel cancer by 50%. The recommendation is that to help reduce the risk of cancer, people should aim for 30 minutes of moderate intensity physical activity at least three times a week.

19 Get physical with the following bite-size 30 minute exercise tips:
- Wash and wax your car.
- Take the dog for a walk.
- Get out in the garden – do your weeding or rake the leaves.
- Walk or cycle to work rather than get in the car again.
- Go for a bike ride with your family or friends.
- Go for a swim.
- Take the stairs rather than the lift at work or in the shopping centre.
- Roll your sleeves up and get dirty with the housework – washing the windows or doing the vacuuming can be quite physical.

Screening

20 There is a pilot NHS Bowel Cancer Screening Programme in progress – see the Reference section at the back of this manual for details.

Being referred for hospital investigation

21 How you are investigated depends on what is available at your local hospital.

22 People with higher risk symptoms should be referred within two weeks for investigation. Most people with these symptoms do not have cancer, but it should be ruled out by special tests.

23 Most diagnostic clinics are run by specialist nurses and doctors. There are

High fibre food	Lower fibre food
Whole grain breads, eg, 100% whole wheat, cracked wheat, multigrain, pumpernickel or dark rye	White bread
Whole grain cereal containing bran, oatmeal, barley, bulgar, cracked wheat; also Shredded Wheat, multigrain or granola cereals	Refined cereals
Whole grain flours, eg, whole wheat, rye, graham (eg, biscuits, muffins)	Foods made with white flour
Whole grain pastas, brown rice or wild rice	Refined pastas, instant or polished rice
Fresh fruits and veg	Fruit juice
Salads (with variety of raw vegetables)	Plain lettuce salads
Baked beans, cooked lentils, split peas	Meat, fish, poultry
Nuts, popcorn, seeds, dried fruit	Crisps, other snacks

a number of different investigations available:
- Flexible sigmoidoscopy – a thin flexible tube with a camera light on the end which can look inside the first 60cms of the bowel.
- Colonoscopy – a long flexible tube to look inside the whole bowel. Laxatives are taken beforehand and no food is taken the day before to empty the bowel. The investigation is usually carried out under sedation.
- Barium enema – a special X-ray examination. A mixture of barium (a thick white liquid which shows up on x-ray) and air is introduced through a tube. Any abnormal areas show up black against the white liquid.

24 The results of the tests are received by the patient at the hospital. Waiting for the results can be worrying and frustrating – and going to the appointment for your news can be extremely nerve-wracking. If you are worried, talk to your family, friends or your GP.

25 If your results are negative, you may be diagnosed with another common gut condition (see *What's Wrong With Me?* above) and given appropriate treatment.

Bowel cancer is not caused by sitting on hot radiators, eating vindaloo or even using newspaper for bog roll.

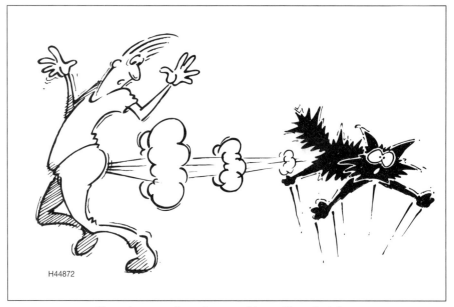

H44872

Bowel cancer is not caused by eating vindaloo

After the diagnosis

26 After initial diagnosis, you will discuss the options open to you with your specialist who will put together a treatment plan (depending on the type and size of the cancer, what stage the cancer is at and your personal health and age) including:

- When and where treatment will take place.
- What drugs will be available.
- Who will be treating you.

27 The main forms of treatment for bowel cancer are as follows.

Surgery

28 During the operation the piece of bowel that contains the cancer is removed and the two open ends are joined together. The lymph nodes near the bowel may also be removed because this is the first place to which the cancer may spread. Surgery can be used alone, or in combination with radiotherapy and/or chemotherapy.

Chemotherapy

29 This treatment uses anti-cancer drugs to destroy the cancer cells and is often given after surgery to reduce the chances of the cancer coming back. It is also given when the cancer is advanced and has spread to other parts of the body.

30 Chemotherapy drugs cause different side effects in different people. Some people experience few side effects; even those who do will have them only temporarily during treatment. Some of the common side effects are tiredness, hair loss, mouth ulcers and nausea. Chemotherapy is sometimes given with radiotherapy before surgery.

Radiotherapy

31 This treatment is normally used only to treat cancer of the rectum and can be given before or after surgery. Radiotherapy may also be given as a palliative treatment to relieve symptoms of the disease, eg, to reduce pain.

Colostomy

32 Most people diagnosed with bowel cancer do not need a colostomy – also called a stoma. Some people may need a temporary stoma but this can often be reversed after a few months. Although people need to time to adjust to having a stoma, life can carry on as normal. Contact the British Colostomy Association for more information.

Will the cancer come back?

33 After you have had treatment, you will need to have regular check-ups every few months to make sure that the cancer has not returned or spread. If the bowel cancer was diagnosed and treated early there is a very good chance that it will not recur after treatment.

34 Even if the cancer does recur it can be treated with a combination of further surgery, chemotherapy or radiotherapy. If the cancer has not returned after five years, you are considered clear.

Emotional support

35 Remaining positive and strong for friends, family and children can be difficult when you are going through the trauma of diagnosis and treatment yourself. Talking to friends or partners can help – but you may also want to ask your doctor about specialist support available to you such as counsellors or nurses.

36 There are also many national and local charities, patient support groups and help lines which could offer you information, help and emotional support. See further information for details.

37 If you can't find the help you need – or want to try to help others – you may want to consider setting up your own local patient support group.

Further information

38 If you would like to know more, look at the contacts section at the back of this book, or contact:

British Colostomy Association
Support, reassurance and practical information for people with a colostomy.
Helpline: 0800 328 4257
Tel: 0118 939 1537
Fax: 0118 923 9184
sue@bcass.org.uk
www.bcass.org.uk

National Association for Colitis and Crohn's Disease (NACC)
Tel: 0845 130 223
NACC in-Contact Support Line:
0845 130 3344
nacc@nacc.org.uk
www.nacc.org.uk

Digestive Disorders Foundation
Tel: 020 7486 0341
ddf@digestivedisorders.org.uk
www.digestivedisorders.org.uk

Ileostomy and Internal Pouch Support Group
Tel: 0800 018 4724
la@ileostomypouch.demon.co.uk
www.ileostomypouch.demon.co.uk

Beating Bowel Cancer
Beating Bowel Cancer is a national charity set up in 1999 to raise awareness of symptoms, promote early diagnosis and encourage open access to treatment choice for those affected by bowel cancer. We encourage people to talk frankly about all aspects of the disease and through our work we aim to save lives from this common cancer.

Current available information
Bowel cancer: The Bottom Line (booklet)
Don't Sit on Your Symptoms (leaflet)
Lifting the Lid on Bowel Cancer (booklet – launched Jan 2004)
Tel: 020 8892 5256
info@beatingbowelcancer.org
www.beatingbowelcancer.org

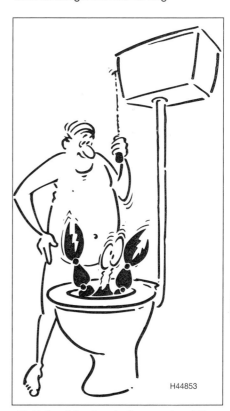

H44853

Talk frankly about all aspects of the disease

6

Some things we do know increase your risk, but the definite cause is still a mystery:

A junk food diet (high in fats and sugars, low in fibre).

Bowel cancer in the close family.

Lack of activity.

Being overweight.

Smoking tobacco.

A bowel condition called polyps or adenomatous polyposis significantly increases your risk, even in another member of your family. Trying to pronounce it can be pretty stressful too.

The good news is you can reduce your risk, even if it is in the family, as follows:

Check out your diet. Reduce the amount of fat and sugars and boost fruit and vegetables.

Regular physical activity and keeping your weight under control.

Discuss any family history with your doctor, who may advise more frequent tests.

Quit the weed! (see Chapter 3).

2 Cancer of the larynx

Introduction

1 Popularly known as the Adam's Apple, the larynx is the box-like structure at the top of the windpipe. Partly composed of gristle (cartilage) it has a prominent front part, especially in men. It has two important jobs: making noise with the vocal cords for the mouth and tongue to turn into speech, and stopping food going down 'the wrong way'. Trying to do both at the same time is one of the tricky bits which can go wrong, especially after a few pints of lager and faced with large chunks of poorly-chewed steak. It has sensitive nerves which make you cough when spaghetti bolognese is boldly going where air should go.

2 Although relatively rare, cancer of the larynx occurs most often in smokers and heavy drinkers. If the cancer is confined to the vocal cords it causes obvious voice changes and is likely to be diagnosed early. In addition, spread from the vocal cords to other parts is thankfully slow. In this case the outlook is favourable. Unfortunately, cancer elsewhere in the larynx is likely to be well advanced before symptoms of breathing or swallowing difficulty arise, so the prospects of a cure is not so good.

Symptoms

3 An obvious symptom of cancer of the larynx is a change in the voice. This is not the usual sore throat of an infection or after speaking for long periods. Singers and actors know this feeling well. With cancer there is a permanent hoarseness. With a longer-standing cancer there can be difficulty in breathing and swallowing.

Causes

4 Tobacco smoking is the single greatest cause, but others include alcohol abuse and exposure to asbestos fibres. Obviously stopping smoking, drinking in moderation and using mixers rather than drinking neat spirits makes sense.

Diagnosis

5 Any marked change in the voice lasting more than a couple of weeks should be investigated by an expert without delay. It is possible to look at the inside of the larynx using an instrument called a fibre optic laryngoscope and any cancer present is generally readily visible.

Prevention

6 As mentioned above, laryngeal cancer is almost totally preventable by stopping smoking, drinking in moderation and avoiding neat spirits.

Treatment

7 Early diagnosis is essential as small cancers of the vocal cords can often be cured by local treatment with lasers, or more often with radiotherapy. Larger cancers that have spread to involve the cartilage of the larynx usually require partial or total removal of the larynx (laryngectomy). Obviously this means the vocal cords are no longer there to vibrate and produce the sounds acted on by the mouth for speech. This is where the latest technology steps in with electromechanical devices that mimic their function. Speech therapists can give invaluable support and advice.

3 Oesophageal (gullet) cancer

Introduction

1 This particularly nasty cancer is unfortunately not rare, with about 1 in 50 of all new cases of cancer being that of the oesophagus. It is more common in people from Iran or China although their risk falls after a few generations in the UK. Men will suffer from this cancer almost twice as often as do women although this is set to change as men increasingly give up smoking, one of the main causes of oesophageal cancer.

2 Although predominantly a disease of old age, men of 45–50 years can develop it As the symptoms tend to be confused with indigestion or heartburn, late presentation to the doctor is the norm rather than the exception.

Cause

3 Drinking neat spirits and smoking come high on the list of suspects, but otherwise the causes are not really known. Pre-existing problems with the gullet such as strictures (narrowing) may increase your risk from cancer but it is by no means certain. Even so it is worth keeping an open mind and seeing your doctor if the symptoms become worse.

Symptoms

4 Unfortunately there may be no symptoms until late in the course of the disease. Once established these can include:

- Pain and difficulty swallowing. This starts with solid food but later includes fluids as well.
- Undigested food being brought up after a meal. If the obstruction is large there can also be problems swallowing saliva until this food is brought back up.
- Persistent coughing as a result of food 'going the wrong way' when being brought back up.
- Weight loss and lack of appetite.

Diagnosis

5 A barium swallow can help show any constriction. A radio opaque solution is swallowed while X-rays are taken; this will be followed by endoscopy using flexible telescope to take samples from any tumour seen. The big danger is from it spreading to other parts of the body and a CT or MRI scan may be used to check for these metastases.

Treatment

6 More than with most other cancers a great deal depends on whether there has been any spread. A localised tumour can be removed, but distant spread is much more difficult to treat. Making swallowing easier by using radiotherapy or chemotherapy to reduce the size of the tumour can make remaining life much more bearable.

Prevention

7 Diluting your drinks and taking them in moderation along with stopping smoking are the best ways of reducing your risk.

4 Cancer of the stomach

Introduction

1 Stomach cancer is thankfully on the decline but is more common in men than in women, affecting about 1 in 7,000 each year. It is the sixth commonest of the potentially fatal cancers but rare under the age of 30, becoming commoner with increasing age.

2 There was great concern amongst some health professionals when ranitidine (Zantac), a treatment for reducing stomach acid production, was released from prescription only-status for sale across the pharmacist's counter. Fears that stomach cancer would go undiagnosed with a consequent increase in deaths were unfounded as, for reasons unknown, the reverse occurred.

Symptoms

3 Stomach upsets are common, but stomach cancer is comparatively rare. Perhaps the most disturbing feature of stomach cancer is the difficulty in distinguishing it from the symptoms of stomach or duodenal ulcers. Most men complain of pain high in the abdomen in the angle between the ribs – follow your breast bone down to the soft bit – it is also often relieved by food. Unlike common stomach upsets, the pain refuses to go away on its own. Some men confuse it with angina, especially if they already suffer from a heart condition. The pain, however, is not helped by nitrate sprays or patches.

4 Late detection is the problem. The difficulty of early diagnosis means the cancer is often advanced by the time it is suspected and symptoms may also include swallowing difficulty, loss of weight, nausea and vomiting. Waiting and hoping it will go away is a bad idea.

Causes

5 Although a lack of fruit and vegetables in the diet may have a link, the jury is still out over foods causing stomach cancer. Things that irritate the stomach such as Helicobacter pylori bacteria may be linked with both stomach ulcers and stomach cancer. Similarly, alcohol and cigarette smoking may also increase your risk. Recent research suggests that too much salt in the diet may also be a factor.

6 As people with blood group A are more likely to develop stomach cancer there may be a genetic element in the causation. If there is stomach cancer in the family you should keep an open mind over stomach upsets or pain that refuses to go away. Even so, the fact that your father or brother developed stomach cancer is by no means an indication that you will as well. The number of men developing stomach cancer is falling

anyway and this may be connected with the fall in cigarette smoking. Reducing your risks makes good sense whatever your blood group or family history.

Diagnosis

7 Not surprisingly, diagnosis of stomach cancer can often be later rather than sooner. This is made all the worse by men's tendency to put off going to see their doctor. Clues come from the symptoms you describe to your doctor, and this is usually followed up with direct viewing through a flexible fibre optic instrument (gastroscope) which provides a view of the cancer and allows biopsies to be taken. A barium meal X-ray will show up stomach cancer in 90 per cent of cases. CT, MRI and ultrasound scanning can also be helpful, especially if there is any possibility of spread to other parts of the body.

Prevention

8 Even though stomach cancer is on the decline you can reduce your risks further through common sense steps such as diluting and moderating your alcohol drinks, but most of all by stopping smoking.

9 If there is any family history of stomach cancer or you suffer from intermittent stomach pain, ask your GP to check for the Helicobacter pylori bacteria.

10 Most importantly, see your doctor early rather than later with any symptoms which refuse to go away or which are not helped by simple painkillers or antacids.

Treatment

11 Treatment depends very much on how soon the cancer is diagnosed. Surgical removal of the tumour is possible if it is not too far advanced, and chemotherapy will generally be used to mop up any remaining tumour cells.

Notes

Chapter 7
Pipes and hoses (urogenital systems)

Contents

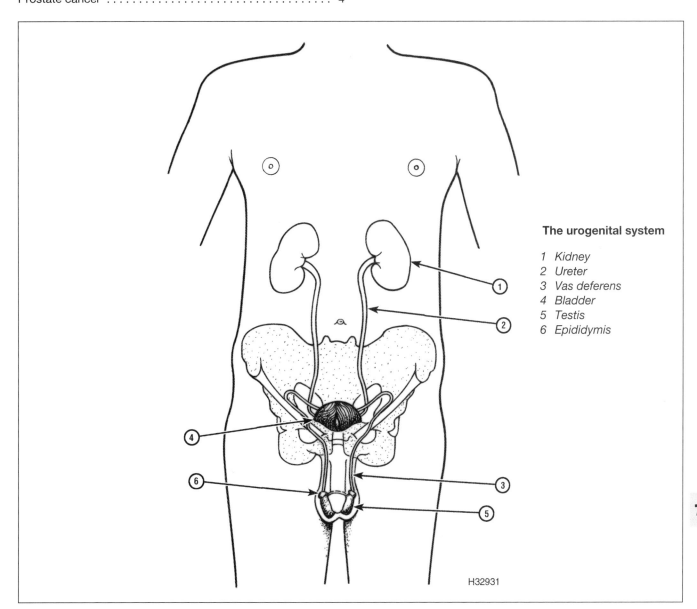

The urogenital system

1 Kidney
2 Ureter
3 Vas deferens
4 Bladder
5 Testis
6 Epididymis

H32931

7

1 Cancer of the bladder

Introduction

1 Bladder cancer accounts for about seven per cent of new male cancers. It is three times as common in men as in women, explained in part by industrial causes where men are the predominant workforce. It is also commoner in white people; the average age at diagnosis is 65. The good news is that the cancer tends to spread slowly, so the majority of tumours are still within the bladder at diagnosis. Even so, early diagnosis improves the chances of survival.

2 A popular misconception is that the bladder is a simple bag to hold urine until a convenient convenience can be found. In fact it is a complex organ with delicate nervous control and intricate muscular layers. We tend to maltreat our bladders terribly, expecting them to do their work without complaint. It is only when things go wrong we realise just how important they are. Sitting low in the pelvis it sits immediately behind the pubic bone. It has three layers, but it is the innermost layer in which cancer generally develops. A full bladder will hold around 350 ml (half a pint) of urine, although some men can seem to store extra in their legs when stood at the bar. Voluntary control is amazingly good and pressures can rise inside the bladder to quite high levels before the point of no return is reached.

3 There is no evidence that constantly holding on causes bladder cancer. Most cancers are caused by carcinogens carried either in the blood or in the urine. Obviously if they are in the urine they can be in contact with the inner layer of the bladder for quite some time, especially overnight. Drinking plenty of fluids helps flush out the carcinogens.

4 If the cancer is detected early and is present only in the innermost layer it can be cured by simple local treatment without opening the bladder (see cystoscopy in *Diagnosis* below). Unfortunately, diagnosis at this stage is not common. After this the cancer will spread into the deeper layers and then eventually outside the bladder itself. Obviously this changes the outcome for successful treatment.

Symptoms

5 Pain is not a major feature of early bladder cancer. Passing blood or pus in the urine are also seen in less serious conditions such as cystitis (bladder infection) but should always be taken seriously, especially when occurring for the first time in older men.

6 If left without early treatment more advanced bladder cancer may cause pain in the flanks (side) or the loins, obstruction to the ureters (the tubes that

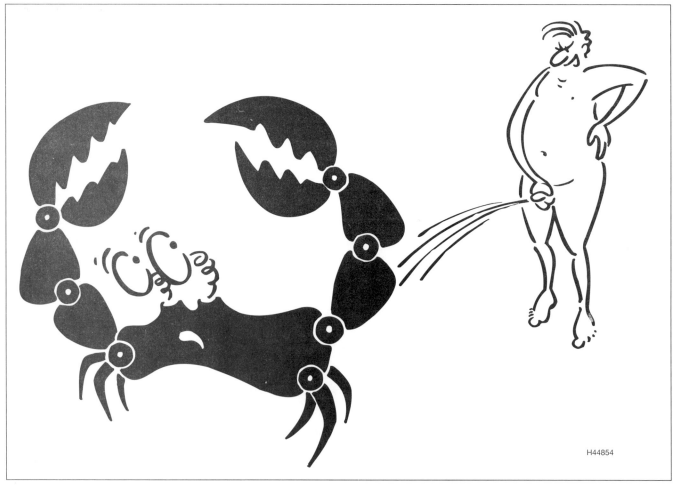

Early diagnosis improves the chances of survival

carry urine down to the bladder from the kidneys), or bone pain from secondary cancer.

Causes

7 Although the causes of most bladder cancers remain uncertain, some of them are known. These include:

- Cigarette smoking (the carcinogens are excreted in the urine). Heavy cigarette smoking is believed to be the cause of half the cases in men.
- Industrial chemicals such as aniline dyes, beta-naphthylamine and benzidine, and chemicals encountered in rubber manufacture (tyre manufacture used to be a major risk).
- Drugs such as phenacetin and cyclophosphamide (paradoxically, used for treating cancer in other parts of the body).
- Possibly long-term bladder inflammation.
- Parasitic disease, especially schistosomiasis (a tropical parasite).
- Possibly the presence of bladder stones.
- Genetic. There is an increased risk if you have bladder cancer in the family. This doesn't automatically mean that you will develop bladder cancer, but you should certainly avoid any triggers such as smoking.

8 Artificial sweeteners, once among the suspects, are now known to be guiltless.

Diagnosis

9 Your symptoms will raise your doctor's suspicions and trigger further examination by specialists.

10 Cystoscopy is examination of the inside of the bladder by means of a fine telescope passed in through the penis (the urethra). You will be delighted to hear that a general anaesthetic is par for the course. Although no-one's idea of a good day out, this enables a distinction to be made between cancers (which are always dangerous) and bladder polyps (which are simply harmless dangly bits within the bladder).

11 As some cells inevitably break off and travel in the urine, this can be examined for the presence of cancer cells.

12 Special X-rays, using a radio-opaque dye that passes through the kidneys into the bladder, may show any tumours inside the bladder.

Prevention

13 Simply stopping smoking and taking proper precautions when using industrial chemicals will prevent most bladder cancers.

Treatment

14 As well as being preventable, bladder cancer is very treatable when caught early. If it is still confined to the inner surface of the bladder, laser treatment or burning with a hot wire (cautery), passed through a cystoscope can be curative. A washout of the bladder with anticancer drugs can also be highly effective, but all need follow up to check for any resurfacing of cancer.

15 Surgery aims to eliminate all cancer, but this is not always possible. In about half of those people presenting with signs of bladder cancer, the tumour is still in the early stages, is confined to the inner lining of the bladder and can readily be destroyed by direct surgery.

16 With spread through the wall of the bladder, major surgery and radiotherapy will be needed. The whole bladder may have to be removed. As with all cancers early detection and prevention is vital.

2 Kidney cancer

Introduction

1 Kidney cancer (or renal carcinoma) now accounts for 3% of all adult tumours. Importantly, the number of new cases diagnosed each year has increased by 30% over the last two decades. Nearly twice as many men than women are affected. The total number of cases however varies considerably from country to country. For example, the rates are relatively low in Asian countries whilst being much higher in North America. The highest rates of all though have been reported in central European countries with nearly 20,000 cases being reported across Europe as a whole last year alone.

2 When compared to other urological cancers, a greater proportion of those diagnosed with this disease will unfortunately die from it. In fact, only 60% of patients with kidney cancer will still be alive 5 years after the diagnosis has been made. Nevertheless, the total number of cases is still very low with only 9 people for every 100,000 of the general population developing the disease each year.

Presenting features

3 For the majority of patients with kidney cancer there are no symptoms until the disease is quite advanced. Often, symptoms appear as a direct result of the size of the tumour and its spread into surrounding structures. About 30% of patients will present to their doctors with evidence of spread of the disease at the time of diagnosis. Blood in the urine, however, may highlight the problem at a much earlier stage and appears in up to 60% of patients. Flank (side) pain is also common and occurs in as many as 40% of those with the disease. A doctor may be able to feel the growth in nearly one-third of patients.

4 Other symptoms appear more vague and range from fatigue and weight loss to night sweats and fever. Some of the symptoms patients experience occur as part of an unusual paraneoplastic syndrome. In these patients the kidney tumour makes hormone-like substances (natural chemical messengers) which result in a wide range of unusual symptoms and signs which can range from sickness and constipation to high blood pressure.

Risk factors

5 Smoking has been consistently linked to developing kidney cancer. The more you smoke, the greater the risk. Importantly, the evidence suggests that this link is strongest of all in men. Being overweight also places the individual at greater risk of developing kidney cancer, as do diets rich in fried and well-cooked meats. Men with a long history of kidney failure and requiring dialysis who develop a cystic disease of the kidney are at greater risk, but there is no good evidence to suggest that there is an association with the more common kidney problems such as kidney stones and infections.

6 There are also a few rare inherited disorders such as the Von Hippel-Lindau (VHL) disease and the Birt-Hogg-Dube syndrome which place affected

7

individuals at greater risk of developing kidney cancer. These however account for only a very small proportion of cases.

Investigations

7 An ultrasound scan of the kidneys is usually one of the first investigations arranged and can detect growths as small as 1 cm in size. In addition to those patients presenting with specific symptoms suggestive of a kidney tumour, many patients will have their diagnosis made by chance whilst undergoing an ultrasound for another problem with which they have consulted their doctor.

8 Frequently a more detailed scan is required to confirm these initial ultrasound findings. This normally involves a CT (computerised tomography) scan. It provides a detailed 'body scan' which can accurately define the extent of the disease and can detect cancers as small as 0.5 cm in size. Unfortunately, the greater sensitivity of these scans means that they can also identify lesions within the kidney which are non-cancerous. Distinguishing between cancerous and non-cancerous lumps on the scan is not always possible and occasionally patients will therefore have operations to take out small masses in the kidney which ultimately turn out to be benign.

9 The management of some of these difficult cases is often helped by magnetic resonance imaging (MRI scanning) which may help in the diagnosis. MRI, however, is more frequently used in patients who have poor kidney function or who have allergies to some of the injectable dyes used with conventional CT scanning. It is extremely accurate and is especially helpful in detecting the extension of a kidney tumour into vein which drains the affected kidney.

Treatment

10 The best treatment is really prevention. Efforts should focus on stopping smoking and encouraging men to attain and then maintain ideal body weights. Additionally, following a diet containing a good proportion of fruit, vegetables and grain along with a reduction in fat would seem the best and easiest way of reducing the risk of developing the disease.

11 Where the disease is present and localised to the kidney, the best treatment is surgery to remove the growth. It remains the only available treatment with the potential for effecting long term cure. Radical nephrectomy involves removing the entire kidney and its surrounding fat. Smaller tumours may be amenable to partial nephrectomy, where a proportion of the healthy kidney is left behind with only the diseased part of the kidney (with a rim of normal tissue) being removed. Only small tumours are amenable to this form of surgery. Some centres may now perform surgery laparoscopically (key-hole surgery) and this type of operation is likely to become more widespread.

12 Where there has been distant spread of the disease outside and away from the kidney, surgery is seldom curative. Unfortunately kidney cancer in these cases does not respond well to chemotherapy either. Instead, greater effort has been directed at boosting the immune system of patients with widespread disease with agents such as interferon and interleukin-2. Whilst these agents give better responses than traditional chemotherapy, the results are still, at best, modest.

13 Newer treatments are currently under investigation (and show some promise), but it is fair to say that disease which is not curable by surgery alone is rarely cured by any of these other measures.

---

3 Cancer of the penis

Introduction

1 Cancer of the penis is rare in this country but is an increasingly important health issue for men in Africa and South America. It accounts for 0.5% of all malignancies amongst men in the UK and Europe and nearly 10% amongst men in Africa. Approximately 400 cases were diagnosed in the UK last year. Whilst it is predominantly a disease of older men (the incidence rising sharply in the sixth decade of life), it is not unusual to find the disease in younger men. Nearly one-quarter of cases have been reported in men less than 40 years of age. Up to 80% of patients with early

disease are still alive and well five years after the diagnosis, but where the disease has spread beyond the penis, less than half will survive that long. There were 100 deaths from penile cancer last year in this country.

Presenting features

2 The first sign of disease is usually a painless warty growth, nodule or an ulcer which appears either on the glans or the foreskin. Frequently these changes are associated with an infection. Nearly half the patients will have an associated phimosis or narrowing in the foreskin such that retraction of the foreskin over the glans is difficult and frequently delays identification and treatment. Eventually, an offensive discharge (sometimes associated with bleeding) prompts the individual to take action. Most of these changes occur on the glans, foreskin or the groove between the two. Very rarely do growths appear on the shaft of the penis itself.

3 When there has been local spread of the disease, patients may present with a lump in the groin which may discharge, ulcerate or bleed. Despite these symptoms and signs it has been estimated that half delay seeking medical treatment for up to one year. Surprising perhaps for a disease involving something that is handled daily!

Risk factors

4 The risk of developing penile cancer appears to be related to a number of factors which include smoking, genital hygiene, and infection with the sexually transmitted human papilloma virus (HPV).

5 The lowest rates of penile cancer are amongst those who have been circumcised. The protective effect appears most marked amongst those circumcised early in life with less marked protective effects being demonstrated amongst those undergoing surgery in adolescence or in adulthood. It would appear that a non-retractile foreskin allows the build-up of smegma (the product of a bacterial action on dead skin cells) which, over a long period of time, can predispose men to penile cancer. Hygiene is therefore essential to reducing the risk of developing the cancer. Importantly, countries where there are low levels of circumcision but good levels of hygiene (such as Denmark) have a low incidence of penile cancer.

6 The greater number of sexual partners that an individual has had, the greater the chance of penile cancer. This appears related to the risk of developing an HPV infection – a virus which has been detected in the tumours of men with penile cancer. Smoking appears to act in concert with this virus to increase the risks even further, so is especially risky for those with this viral infection.

Investigations

7 A biopsy of the growth is the single most important investigation. It not only confirms the diagnosis but also assesses the aggressiveness of the disease and the likelihood of it having spread beyond the confines of the penis. A circumcision or longitudinal incision in the foreskin is often necessary to allow the biopsy to be performed. For small growths there is little need for further investigation.

8 Where the growth is thought to have invaded much deeper into the penis, an ultrasound or MRI scan may prove useful in determining the extent and nature of any planned surgery. A CT scan is often used to look for distant spread of the disease – most commonly identified in lymph nodes located in the groin area.

Treatment

9 If the cancer is confined to the foreskin then circumcision may be all that is required to treat the disease. Those with very superficial cancers involving the glans may be successfully treated with laser treatment, radiotherapy or a surgical technique known as Mohs microresection. All of these are designed to leave the bulk of the penis intact. Those with deeper penetrating tumours require more extensive surgery, which may involve a partial or total amputation of the penis, or radiotherapy. The best success rates are reported when at least 2 cm of healthy tissue are taken in addition to the diseased area because it reduces the chances of the disease returning.

10 Involvement of the lymph nodes in one or both groins is an important feature of the disease and has a direct bearing on the success rate of treatments. Many patients, however, will have an associated infection which can

also cause swellings in the groin. After initial treatment of the penis therefore, those patients with groin swellings are treated with antibiotics for several weeks. Those who have a persistent swelling despite this require surgery to remove the lymph nodes. If there is disease within these glands then surgery on the other groin is also necessary, as nearly half of these individuals will be found to have disease there too, even if no swellings can be felt. Some patients who have aggressive forms of the disease may require groin surgery (even if no swelling is ever demonstrated) to improve their chances of making a complete recovery.

11 For patients who have disease which has spread beyond the penis and groins there are few treatment options. Whilst there have been some complete cures in a minority of such patients with radiotherapy, radiotherapy combined with chemotherapy or even occasionally with chemotherapy alone, such cures are rare. Treatment of these rare cases is centralised to get the best combination of surgeon, radiotherapist and medical oncologist with adequate experience in their management.

---

4 Prostate cancer

What is the prostate gland and what does it do?

1 Only men have a prostate gland. It's roundish and about the size of a golf ball. It is in the pelvis, hard up against the base of the bladder. The prostate surrounds the urethra – the tube that runs from your bladder inside your penis to the outside. You pee through it. Imagine the prostate as a fat rubber washer round a bit of tubing and you'll get the picture.

2 It grows to adult size at puberty, under the influence of hormones. In most men it also begins to enlarge again in early middle age. An enlarged prostate can cause problems for older men when they pee. These prostate problems are common.

3 The prostate's main job is to make prostatic fluid, one of four different fluids of the liquid part of semen. (Semen

carries sperm and is what you ejaculate when you have an orgasm.) The prostate gland is, in fact, made up of a mass of smaller secretory glands which make prostatic fluid. It is also made of muscle, which contracts at orgasm expelling the fluid into the penis. This contraction contributes to some of the 'push' of ejaculation.

Prostate cancer is not caused by vasectomy, injury, masturbation or reading the Kama Sutra under the bedclothes with a torch. Just as well or it could be teenagers suffering along with men predominately aged over 50.

When things go wrong

4 Problems with the prostate are common. Because of where the prostate is, peeing can become more difficult.

5 The kind of symptoms you might have due to a prostate problem are:
  a) *A frequent need to urinate especially at night.*
  b) *A need to rush to the toilet so that you may even wet yourself sometimes.*
  c) *Difficulty starting to pass urine.*
  d) *Straining or taking a long time to finish.*
  e) *A weak flow.*
  f) *A feeling that your bladder has not emptied properly.*
  g) *Pain on passing urine.*
  h) *Pain on ejaculation.*
  i) *Pain in the genitals.*

6 Some prostate problems are more serious than others. Prostatitis can affect men at any age and causes pain and discomfort due to inflammation and sometimes infection. BPH, or benign enlargement of the prostate, the most common prostate condition, affects older men. It can be quite uncomfortable. If you are an older man and have urinary symptoms this is the most likely cause. However, prostate cancer is a possibility.

7 If you are concerned about any symptoms you may have, visit your GP. He or she can examine you and decide whether you have no problem, an easily treated problem or a more serious one, like prostate cancer.

7

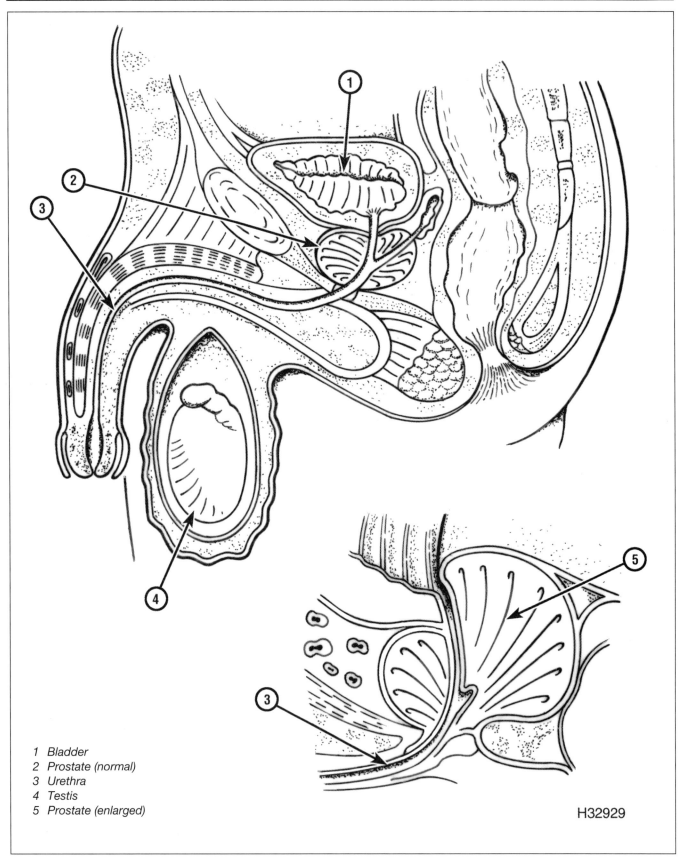

1 Bladder
2 Prostate (normal)
3 Urethra
4 Testis
5 Prostate (enlarged)

H32929

Normal and enlarged prostate gland

Prostate cancer is catching up with skin cancer as the number one male cancer in the UK.

What goes wrong?

8 Normally the growth of all cells in the body is carefully regulated. When cancer develops, the cells multiply and grow in an uncontrolled way and can spread elsewhere in the body.

9 Most commonly, prostate cancer is a slow-growing cancer and it can remain undetected because it never causes problems in a man's lifetime. But this is not true of all men. A few men will have aggressive cancers which spread quickly. Sometimes men have no hint that there is anything wrong until cancer cells move outside the gland and cause symptoms elsewhere in the body, often in bone.

Who gets prostate cancer?

10 Prostate cancer is diagnosed in more than 25,000 men every year in the UK and the number is rising as more cases are being detected due to the increased use of the PSA test (see Reference section at the back of this manual for details). The majority of men diagnosed will be over sixty – commonly in their seventies. Men can be affected from the age of about 45 but this is rare. The risk of getting prostate cancer gets higher as men get older.

11 Older men of African or African Caribbean origin are at particular risk of getting prostate cancer. Men who have had a close male blood relative, particularly a brother, diagnosed with it seem also to have an increased risk of getting it themselves.

12 The Westernised diet of highly refined food with a high animal fat content also seems to increase the risk of developing prostate cancer. There is no firm evidence how to reduce the risk of prostate cancer but we know that adopting a healthy diet with more fruit and vegetables, less red meat and more fish is good for reducing the risks of other cancers and heart disease, and possibly prostate cancer.

What are the symptoms?

13 It is important to be clear: Not all men get symptoms that show they have prostate cancer. In the men that do, not all men have exactly the same symptoms. You do not have to have all the symptoms on the list.

The symptoms are usually related to problems peeing:

  a) Frequent need to urinate, especially at night.
  b) Rushing to the toilet.
  c) Difficulty starting to urinate.
  d) Straining to pass urine.
  e) Taking a long time.
  f) Having a weak flow.
  g) Getting the feeling that your bladder has no emptied properly when you have finished urinating.
  h) Dribbling after urination is complete.
  i) Pain or discomfort on passing urine.

In addition, other symptoms can be:

  j) Lower back pain.
  k) Pain in the pelvis, hips or thighs.
  l) Impotence.
  m) Blood in the urine – but this is rarer.

14 It is important to realise that any of these symptoms are also caused by problems which are nothing to do with prostate cancer. If you are concerned about any symptoms that you have, visit your GP.

Diagnosis at the GP

15 When a GP thinks there might be a prostate problem he or she will do some tests. Common tests are:

16 A blood test to measure the PSA level. Prostate Specific Antigen (PSA) is

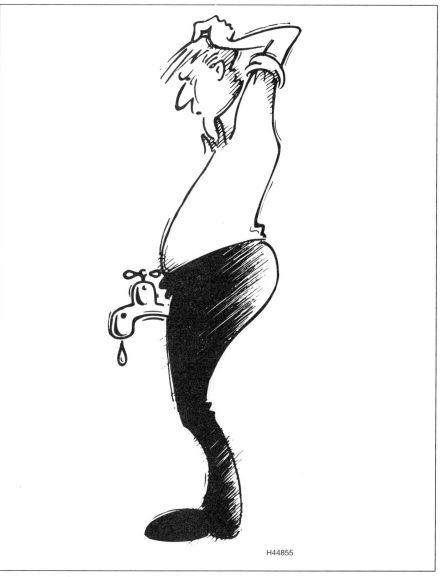

H44855

The symptoms are usually related to problems peeing

a protein that the prostate produces. It is normal for a man to have some PSA in the blood. If there is a problem with the prostate the levels of PSA in the blood can go up. The normal level is up to about 4 for a man of 60. It is slightly less for younger men and slightly more for older men. The PSA test is not a test for cancer, but it can show the GP that there is a problem with the prostate. The PSA test result may show that other tests in hospital are needed.

17 A physical examination called a DRE. A digital rectal examination (DRE) is a simple test done by the GP. The doctor feels your prostate through your rectum, either while you lie on your side or bend over a chair. Some men find a DRE uncomfortable or embarrassing, but it is over quickly.

18 Your doctor may feel an irregularity on the surface of the prostate that makes him suspect cancer. An area may feel harder than the rest, or perhaps knobbly. If he or she has concerns because of the PSA and DRE and any symptoms that you are having he or she will suggest that you go to the hospital for other tests.

You may be able to reduce your risk by taking selenium and vitamin E supplements along with the occasional Bloody Mary, preferably with less Mary. Tomatoes reportedly reduce your risk.

Tests in hospital

19 There will be further tests in hospital. The specialist may suggest that you need a biopsy. This means a sample of tissue is taken from the prostate for analysis. This is done using a TRUS (Trans Rectal Ultra Sound) guided biopsy.

20 The doctor looks at the prostate with an ultrasound probe. This is put into your rectum and images shown on a screen. Local anaesthetic is used to dull pain in the area from which the samples will be taken. The doctor uses the images to guide the sampling needles into the prostate, then removes a small amount of tissue from the gland with the needles.

21 The pathologist (lab specialist) looks at the sample under the microscope. A report of the findings is sent to your urologist. If there is a cancer, the report will say whether it is slow growing, moderately aggressive or aggressive. The pathologist may mention the Gleason score. This is a way of using numbers to show the aggressiveness of the tumour. Two is the least aggressive and ten the most aggressive. It is important for the specialist to know how aggressive the cancer is, because this can affect the treatment options.

22 Other tests may be done. The doctors need to check whether the cancer has moved outside the gland. Like your Gleason score, the results of these tests may change your treatment options.

23 The specialist may suggest a CT scan. CT is a way of using X rays to take images like slices through the body. This allows the doctors to see the prostate, surrounding tissues and lymph nodes.

24 Magnetic Resonance Imaging (MRI) is another way of looking inside the body but does not use X-ray. Powerful magnets are used to make the images.

25 You may also need a bone scan. This depends on your other results. If the prostate cancer has spread some

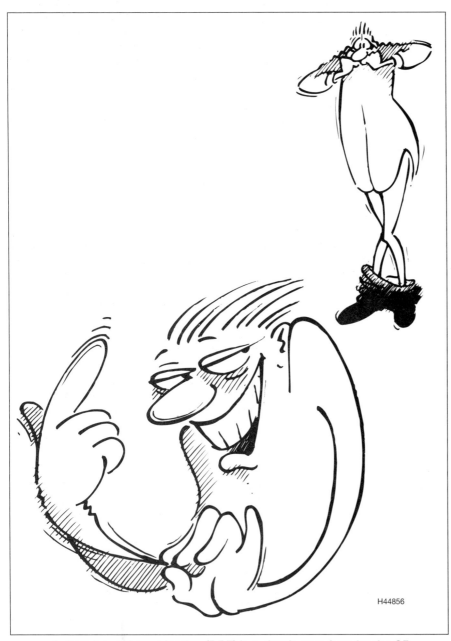
H44856

A digital rectal examination (DRE) is a simple test done by the GP

distance, bone is the most likely place to find it.

Treatment

26 Prostate cancer is treated in several different ways. It depends on how aggressive the cancer is, where the cancer is in your body and how old you are. Your general state of health may make a difference. Treatment will also depend on the choices you decide to make.

27 Your urologist will discuss different options with you. You may see some other specialists such as a medical oncologist (who specialises in the treatment of cancer with medicines) or a radiotherapist, often called a clinical oncologist, who treats cancer using radiation therapy.

Localised cancer

28 If the cancer is localised, that is, only present inside the gland, it can be treated by radiotherapy, brachytherapy or surgery – see below. Your specialist may also discuss the 'no treatment' option – active surveillance – with you.

29 All the treatments have side effects. You need to consider these when choosing treatments. Active surveillance, as explained later, avoids these side effects and might be an option open to you. Impotence and incontinence are the side effects which cause most concern.

30 The treatment options can be hard to decide on, as there is no clear cut 'best treatment' for most men. You may feel at a loss when you are encouraged to decide for yourself if you expect your a doctor to make a clear recommendation. It really will be up to you.

Radiotherapy

31 External beam radiotherapy is widely available and most units will now be offering the modern 3D conformal option. A course of treatment lasts five days a week, for 5–7 weeks. Possible side effects to discuss with a specialist include pain on passing urine, incontinence, bowel problems and impotence. You may be offered additional hormone therapy to help improve your body's response to radiotherapy.

32 Brachytherapy is an internal radiotherapy treatment where radioactive seeds are implanted into the prostate. This is done under anaesthetic

and involves an overnight stay in hospital. Brachytherapy is available in the UK but only at selected centres. Brachytherapy is not suitable for all men. If you are a good candidate for surgery it is also likely that you are a good candidate for brachytherapy. Side effects are mostly urinary problems. Impotence can occur as a longer term effect of this treatment.

33 Cryotherapy is a new treatment. It is not available in every area at the moment, but increasing numbers of centres are offering it. Doctors who do prostate cryotherapy use it for men who have already had radiotherapy as a 'first choice' treatment, but where the prostate cancer has recurred in the same area. Ultra-thin needles are inserted into the prostate through which pressurised freezing gases reach the cancer and treat it by forming a destructive ice-ball. At the time of going to press it is performed at 7 centres in the NHS. Like some other treatments, incontinence is a possible side effect.

Surgery

34 The prostate can also be surgically removed in an operation called a radical prostatectomy. Surgery is not suitable for all men. For example it is not usually offered as an option for men over 70. If you are over 70 and choose radical treatment you are more likely to be offered radiotherapy. Impotence and incontinence are significant risks of this kind of operation. Ask your surgeon for details of how they may affect you later on. Recently radical prostatectomy has become available as a 'keyhole' operation. Only a few surgeons offer this approach but it may become more common in time.

Monitoring

35 As many prostate cancers are slow growing and non aggressive your specialist may suggest active monitoring or surveillance for you. Your PSA level will be cheeked regularly and you may have occasional repeat biopsies. Thus the cancer is monitored rather than treated. This is a good way of avoiding the side effects of treatment when the cancer is causing no physical problems. This option is most commonly recommended for older men. There may be good reasons for you taking this option, especially when your cancer is

slow growing. Do not think your doctors are just saving money! You do not have to choose this option if you are unhappy with it.

Men have roughly the same risk of developing prostate cancer as women have of breast cancer.

Advanced prostate cancer

36 If the cancer has moved beyond the gland, your options are different. The cancer may be locally advanced – that is, in the tissues surrounding the prostate; or advanced – that is, affecting distant parts of your body. An operation to remove the prostate would still leave cancer behind so that is not a choice that will be offered to you. Your doctors may offer you radiotherapy and additional hormone therapy if you have a locally advanced cancer. You may be offered hormone therapy alone. It depends on each individual case.

Hormone therapy

37 Prostate cancer needs the male hormone testosterone to grow and continue spreading. By depriving the cancer of testosterone, hormone therapy can cause the cancer to shrink . It will usually make the PSA levels drop too, to immeasurable levels in some men. Hormone therapy is good for relieving symptoms of the cancer, particularly bone pain and urinary problems. But it is not without side effects itself.

38 Hormone therapy does not cure the cancer but there is an excellent chance that it will keep the cancer in check for several years. It works wherever the cancer is in your body.

39 Drug treatments are commonly used as hormone therapy. This means you will be given monthly or three monthly injections, or daily tablets, or a combination of both. Your doctors will help you decide which treatment is best for you.

40 There is also a surgical from of hormone therapy. The testicles can be removed. With the improved modern drugs which are equally effective, these operations are much less common. It sounds alarming but for some men this is a good option. Such surgery is never performed without your fully informed

7

consent. You do not have to choose this option if you are unhappy with it.

41 Common side effects of all forms of hormone therapy are: hot flushes, problems getting and maintaining erections and loss of interest in sex. Breast tenderness or swelling may also occur.

42 Hormone therapy eventually becomes ineffective against the cancer. Chemotherapy may then be offered. It is not used earlier because all the other treatments outlined here work better. However, at the later stages of prostate cancer chemotherapy works well in keeping the cancer at bay. It will not cure the cancer but should improve quality of life.

Making choices

43 More than with many other conditions, there is no clear 'best treatment' for prostate cancer. Your doctor will explain the options to you, but you have to make the choice. This is not easy when you are having to come to terms with a diagnosis of cancer, so making choices also depends on having the right support around you. Your GP will help you. Your specialists, too – and their teams often includes specialist nurses whose job it is to support and inform you. Your family and friends will also be on your side.

Your sleeping partner might not be. Sleeping, that is.
Your frequent trips to the loo can be disruptive – you have the problem but unfortunately it's your partner who has seen the doctor and is taking the sleeping tablets to treat it.

Further information

If you would like to know more, look at the contacts section at the back of this book, or contact:

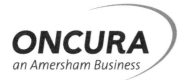

ONCURA
an Amersham Business

The Prostate Cancer Charity
Produces a wide range of literature about prostate cancer which they send

out free of charge. The information is also available on their website. They also provide a confidential helpline staffed by experienced nurses on weekdays and Wednesday evenings. The nurses answer questions from anyone: men who have been diagnosed, the general public, friends or relatives concerned about prostate cancer, the PSA test; any aspects of a healthy lifestyle; coping with a diagnosis. If you have prostate cancer they can also send you out information tailored to your specific needs. Ask about The Tool Kit.

Helpline: 0845 300 8383
www.prostate-cancer.org.uk

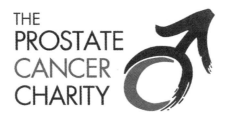

THE
PROSTATE
CANCER
CHARITY

The Orchid Cancer Appeal
Tel: 020 7601 7808
www.orchid-cancer.org.uk

5 Scrotal cancer

Introduction

1 Cancer of the scrotum was first and most famously described by Sir Percival Pott as occurring predominantly amongst chimney sweeps in 1775. It was one of the first descriptions of a tumour which arose as a direct result of chemicals in the environment – in this case chimney soot. Aromatic hydrocarbons in soot, tars and petroleum products are now known to be carcinogens or cancer-causing agents. The tumours are very rare today. In addition to the commonest form of the disease (squamous cell carcinoma) there are a number of rarer varieties which have not been linked with industrial chemicals.

Presenting features

2 An ulcer or wart like growth may be the first sign of the disease. It may bleed or become infected. In time the growth

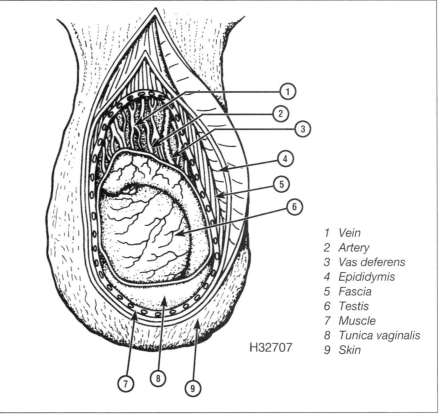

1 Vein
2 Artery
3 Vas deferens
4 Epididymis
5 Fascia
6 Testis
7 Muscle
8 Tunica vaginalis
9 Skin

H32707

Testis and scrotum

may spread to the groin where a lump may be felt.

Risk factors

3 Exposure to environmental carcinogens was classically associated with 'chimney sweeps' and 'mule spinners' in years gone past. In the western world such presentations are rare today. They may still be implicated however in many parts of the developing world.

Diagnosis

4 A biopsy of the growth is the most important investigation. A CT (body scan) may be used to assess whether the tumour has spread to other parts of the body.

Treatment

5 Surgery to remove the growth is the treatment of choice. Taking a good rim of normal tissue reduces the risk of it recurring in the same area. The underlying testicle is very rarely involved and so does not need to be removed. When there has been spread to the glands in the groin these need to be removed as well. Where there has been spread to other parts of the body, chemotherapy or radiotherapy may help control the symptoms of the disease but is rarely curative.

---

6 Testicular cancer

The Orchid Cancer Appeal would like to thank CancerBACUP for their assistance with this section.

What are the testicles and what do they do?

1 The testicles are two small oval-shaped organs (they can also be called testes or gonads), and are the male sex glands. They are located behind the penis in a pouch of skin called the scrotum. The testicles produce sperm and testosterone. The testicles are located outside the body because sperm develop best at a temperature several degrees cooler than normal internal body temperature.

2 The germ cells inside the seminiferous tubules create sperm. The sperm move into the epididymis where they mature. They are stored there for a

few weeks until they eventually move up the vas deferens to combine with fluids from the prostate and seminal vesicles to form what you normally think of as semen. The whole process takes about seven weeks.

3 The Leydig cells distributed throughout the testicle are the body's main source of testosterone. Testosterone, the male sex hormone, is essential to the development of the reproductive organs and other male characteristics such as:

• Body and facial hair.
• Low voice.
• Muscle development.
• The ability to have an erection.
• Sex drive (libido).

4 Without enough testosterone, a man

may lose his sex drive and suffer from fatigue, depression, hot flushes and osteoporosis (thinning of the bones).

What causes testicular cancer?

5 The exact causes of testicular cancers are as yet unknown. In the unborn child testicles develop inside the abdomen between the kidneys, and then descend into the scrotum at birth or in the first year of life. Testicular cancer is known to be more common in men who have had a testicle which has failed to descend. Also a man has a four times higher risk of developing testicular cancer if his father has been diagnosed with the disease, or eight times the risk if a brother has been diagnosed with the disease. A sedentary lifestyle can

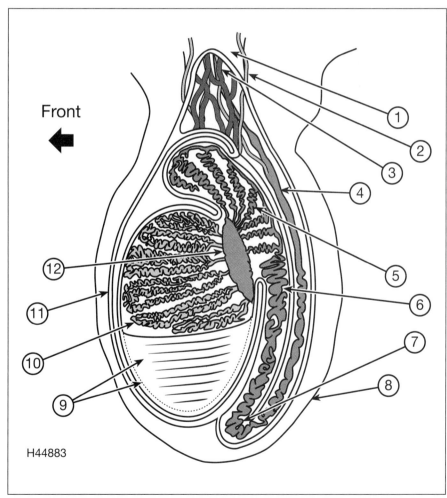

H44883

Cross-section of testis

1 Spermatic cord	5 Epididymis head	9 Tunica albuginea
2 Blood vessels	6 Epididymis body	10 Seminiferous tubules
3 Veins	7 Epididymis tail	11 Tunica vaginalis
4 Ductus deferens	8 Skin	12 Rete testis

7

increase risk but regular exercise can reduce it.

6 There is no proven link between injury or sporting strains (eg, being hit in the testes by a football) and testicular cancer. There is some evidence to suggest that an increase in hormone levels after an injury may accelerate precancerous changes. However, more significantly, an injury can produce a swelling, which may mask a tumour.

The risk

7 Testicular cancer, though the most common cancer in young men, is rare. Overall there are around 2,000 cases diagnosed each year in the UK. The lifetime risk for being diagnosed with testicular cancer is one in 259. The highest at risk age group is between 18–32 years old. There has been an 84% rise in incidence of testicular cancer in Britain since the late 1970s and this rate is still increasing. As testicular cancer can usually be successfully treated, mortality is very low. Advances in the treatment of testicular cancer has led to a fall in UK mortality rates since the late 1970s, the mortality rate is now only 0.3 per 100,000.

8 In more than one third of cases the

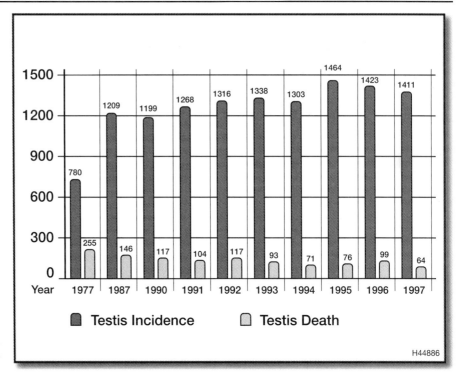

Changing incidence and death rates of testicular cancer in England and Wales

cancer has already spread by the time of diagnosis. Despite this, today more than 95% of patients are cured, albeit many needing toxic drug treatment

(chemotherapy). If caught at an early stage, the treatment is much more simple and may only require surgery to the diseased testicle; the cure rate at this stage is more than 99%. Surveys suggest that many men are unaware of testicular cancer or prefer to ignore it and only 5% of men regularly check their testicles. A simple regular check-up is now known to help detect the early signs and reduce the amount of treatment needed.

The symptoms of testicular cancer

9 The most common symptoms are a swelling or a small lump on the side of a testicle. There may also be an ache in the lower abdomen or in the affected testicle although this is quiet rare. In a few men the testicle may suddenly become swollen and very tender.

10 A few patients who have very small tumours, occasionally may be diagnosed because they become generally unwell, possibly with night sweats, loss of appetite, weight loss, stomach ache, back ache, a cough or tenderness in the breast due to the tumour spreading outside the testicle.

11 It is because of these cases that

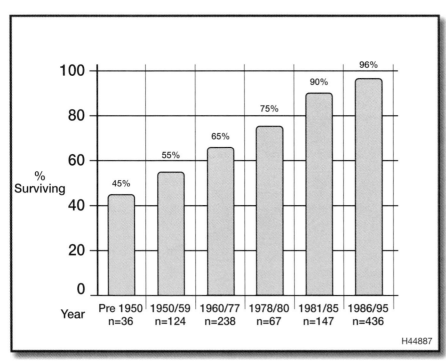

The change in ten-year survival of all patients with testis tumour at the Royal London Hospitals

doctors should routinely check the testicle as part of a routine examination of the abdomen.

12 None of the above symptoms necessarily mean that you have testicular cancer, but if you do find a swelling in a testicle or any other symptom it is important to go to a GP as soon as possible to be checked over.

Testicular self examination

13 From the time of puberty onwards, it is important that all men are aware of what is normal for themselves (there are slight differences in everybody). It is picking up changes such as areas of hardening or swelling that indicate a need to do something.

14 The best time to check your testicles is in a warm bath or shower, as the muscles of the scrotal sac are more relaxed. Cradle the scrotum in the palm of both hands and use the thumb and fingers to gently squeeze the testicles, one at a time (see Chapter 4, Section 3). Learn to differentiate between the main body and the epididymis collecting tubes. Lumps in the collecting tubes are relatively common and almost invariably benign. Lumps in the body are rarer but more important and need to be acted on quickly. One testicle may hang lower than the other and be different in size and even have areas of discomfort without having testicular cancer. The critical issue is looking for changes in consistency and areas of hardening and swelling, which are usually painless.

Different types of testicular cancer

15 Most lumps in the testicles are benign cysts, which are caused by a blockage in one of the tubes, these are not cancer. They do not spread to other parts of the body and are seldom a threat to life. Benign tumours can be removed by surgery if they become large and/or uncomfortable, and they are not likely to return. Malignant tumours (cancers) can invade and destroy nearby healthy tissues and organs. Cancerous cells can also spread to other parts of the body and form new tumours.

16 The two main types of testicular cancer are called seminomas and teratomas. These tumours are also known as Germ Cell Cancers as they develop in germ cells within the testis.

Seminomas account for about 40 percent of all testicular cancer. Usually, seminomas are slow-growing and tend to stay localised in the testicle for long periods and occur in men between 25 and 55 years of age. Teratomas usually affect a younger group of men from 15 to 35 years old and tend to be more aggressive than seminomas. Less commonly, cancers can develop within other cells within the testis, these are known as Non-Germ Cell Cancers.

Diagnosis by the GP

17 Usually you begin by seeing your GP who will examine you and take your medical details. He or she will then refer you to a hospital specialist for further tests, expert advice and treatment.

Referral to a specialist

18 The specialist will give you a full physical examination and take your medical history. You may have a special ultrasound test of the scrotum and the

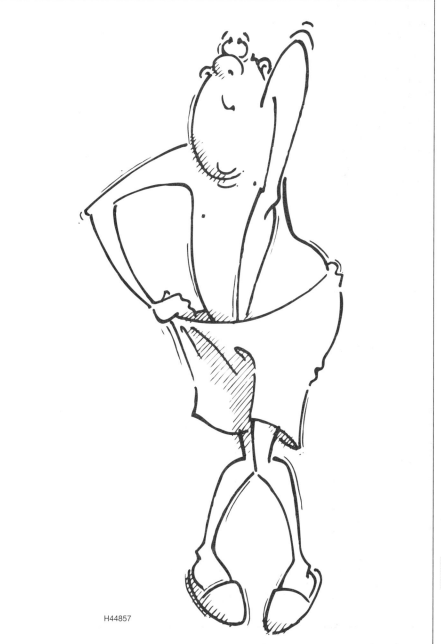

Use the thumb and fingers to gently squeeze the testicles

7

testes. This test can often distinguish between cancer and lumps due to other causes. It uses sound waves to build up a picture of the testes and scrotum. The test is painless and occurs on the skin surface. However, the only way to confirm that the swelling is cancer is for a surgeon to examine the testicle during an operation. During the surgery the surgeon can usually see whether the lump is a cancer or not. Sometimes a small piece of tissue is removed and immediately examined under a microscope by a pathologist (this is known as a biopsy). If the biopsy shows that the lump is a cancer the testicle will be removed (this operation is known as orchidectomy, and the procedure is via an abdominal excision, and not through the scrotal sac).

19 The cells are then taken to the laboratory and examined further to find out which type of testicular cancer it is.

20 You can usually go home the next day. If the cancer has not spread beyond the testicle, this may be the only treatment you need, although for a few years you will have to attend the hospital regularly as an outpatient for check-ups.

21 The removal of one testicle does not affect your ability to have an erection or to father children. An artificial testicle (known as an implant or prosthesis) can be inserted into your scrotum to restore a normal appearance. The specialist will be able to give more details.

Further tests

22 If the tests show that you do have testicular cancer, your doctor will want you to have some further tests to see if there has been any spread of the cancer to other parts of the body.

23 These tests may include some or all of the following:
- Blood tests.
- Chest X-ray and CT scan (CAT scan).
- Magnetic resonance imaging (MRI or NMR scan).
- Positron Emission Tomography scan (PET Scan).
- Blood tests.

24 Some testicular cancers produce chemicals which are released into the bloodstream. The two main chemicals, called markers, are alpha-fetoprotein (AFP) and beta human chorionic gonadotrophin (BHCG). If they are present in the blood, they can be used to measure the effect of treatment on the cancer.

25 Samples of your blood will also be taken regularly throughout your treatment to check your general health and the effect that any treatment may be having on the normal cells in your blood.

Chest X-ray and CT scan (CAT scan)

26 Usually a chest X-ray or CT scan are done to check for any signs that the cancer has spread to your lungs or to the lymph glands in your abdomen The CT scan takes a series of X-rays which are fed into a computer to build up a three-dimensional picture of the inside of the body. The scan takes from 10 to 30 minutes. You may be given a drink or injection of a dye which allows particular areas to be seen more clearly. For a few minutes, this may make you feel hot all over. If you are allergic to iodine or have asthma you could have a more serious reaction to the injection, so it is important to let your doctor know beforehand. You will probably be able to go home as soon as the scan is over. The scan is painless but it will mean lying still for 10–30 minutes

Magnetic resonance imaging (MRI or NMR scan)

27 This test uses magnetism to build up cross-sectional pictures of your body. Some people are given an injection of dye into a vein in the arm to improve the image.

28 During the scan you will be asked to lie very still on a couch inside a long chamber for up to an hour. This can be unpleasant if you don't like enclosed spaces; if so, it may help to mention this to the radiographer. The MRI scanning process is also very noisy, but you will be given earplugs. You can usually take someone with you into the room to keep you company.

29 The chamber is a very powerful magnet, so before entering the room you should remove any metal belongings. People who have cardiac monitors, pacemakers or metal surgical clips cannot have an MRI scan because of the magnetic fields.

Positron Emission Tomography scan (PET Scan)

30 PET scans are a new type of scan and you may have to travel to a specialist centre to have one. They are not always necessary but you can discuss with your doctor whether one would be useful in your case. PET scans can be used to find whether testicular cancer has spread beyond the testes, or to examine any lumps that remain after treatment to see whether they are scar tissue, or whether cancer cells are still present.

31 A PET scan uses low-dose radioactive sugar to measure the activity of cells in different parts of the body. A very small amount of a mildly radioactive substance is injected into a vein, usually in your arm. A scan is then taken. Areas of cancer are usually more active than surrounding tissue and show up on the scan.

32 Once you have had all the tests you need, the doctor will have a good idea of the type of cancer and the stage (whether it is just within the testicle or has spread). It will probably take several days for the results of your tests to be ready and a follow-up appointment will be made for you.

Staging of testicular cancer

33 The stage of a cancer is a term used to describe its size and whether it has spread beyond its original site. There are several staging systems for testicular cancer. Generally it is divided into four stages, from small and localised (stage one), to spread into surrounding structures or other parts of the body (stage four). Knowing the extent of the cancer and the type of cell involved helps the doctors decide on the most appropriate treatment.

34 The staging system most commonly used in the UK is described below.

35 Tumour in situ (TIS): this is when there are a small number of cancer cells which are completely contained within the lining of the collecting tubules in the testicle. TIS is sometimes referred to as precancerous changes. Subsequent stages are:
- Stage one tumours: these are completely contained within the testicle.
- Stage two tumours: the cancer cells have spread to the lymph nodes in the pelvic area or the back of the abdomen.
- Stage three tumours: there are cancer cells present in the lymph nodes in the chest or above the collarbones.

- Stage four tumours: these have spread into other organs. The most common place is the lung.

Types of treatment

36 Treatment for testicular cancer is usually very successful and most men can now be completely cured, even if the cancer has spread beyond the testicles. The treatment will depend on the type of cancer (whether it is a teratoma or a seminoma) and whether it has spread beyond the testes.

37 There are three main types of treatment:

- Surgery.
- Radiotherapy.
- Chemotherapy.

Surgery

38 Surgical removal of the testicle (orchidectomy) is usually the first treatment for both seminoma and teratoma. It also enables your doctor to make an exact diagnosis. But remember, no operation or procedure will be carried out without your written consent.

39 It is uncommon for cancer to affect both testicles. A very small proportion of men develop a new cancer in the remaining testicle. For this reason a small biopsy of the unaffected testicle may be suggested at the time of the initial orchidectomy or during follow-up. This is a procedure in which a thin needle is passed through the skin of the scrotum to take a small sample of cells from the testicle. If no signs of early cancer are present this is very reassuring. If the earliest stage of cancer is present (carcinoma in situ) this can be cured by a low dose of radiotherapy.

40 Further surgery is sometimes needed after radiotherapy or chemotherapy, to remove any cancer cells that may still be in the lymph glands of the abdomen or chest.

Further treatment

41 If the cancer has not spread and was completely removed with the testicle, the operation may be the only treatment you will need.

Surveillance

42 After your operation, it is very important for you to be seen regularly in the outpatients clinic by your doctor for blood tests, chest X-rays and CT scans. This is because in some patients the cancer may come back in the glands at the back of the abdomen or in the lungs. If your doctor feels that the risk of the cancer returning is very low, you will be seen regularly in the clinic and will not have any further treatment unless your tests show that the cancer has come back. This is known as a surveillance policy. In the small proportion of men in whom the cancer does come back, the

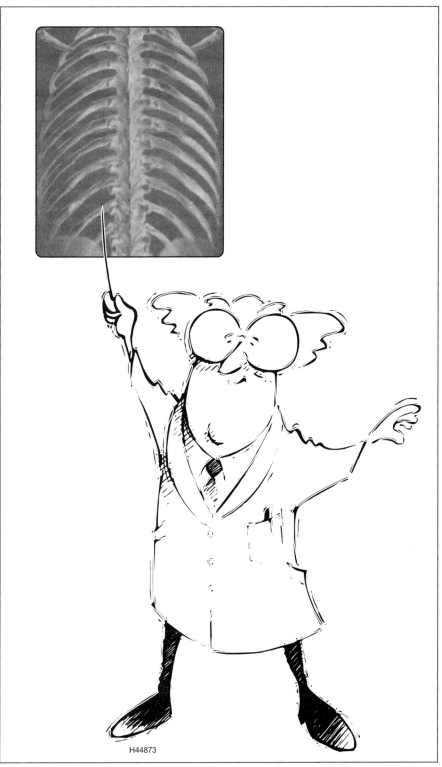

H44873

It is very important for you to be seen regularly for chest X-rays

7

regular tests will detect the cancer when it is still very small and further treatment can give an excellent chance of cure.

43 If the risk of the cancer returning is thought to be higher, it may be necessary to give further treatment to prevent this happening. This is known as adjuvant therapy and the type of treatment will depend on the type of cancer:

Teratoma

44 Teratoma is very sensitive to chemotherapy. If the teratoma seemed to be contained within the testicle, two courses of chemotherapy may be given following orchidectomy, to reduce the chance of recurrence. Three or four courses of chemotherapy may be given if the teratoma has spread beyond the testicle, or if it comes back after orchidectomy.

Seminoma

45 Even if the seminoma has not spread, men may be offered surgery, followed by radiotherapy to the glands at the back of the abdomen, to reduce the chance of recurrence. A single dose of chemotherapy is being tried as an alternative to this treatment. Radiotherapy will be given if the seminoma has spread to the lymph glands at the back of the abdomen. If the lymph glands are large or if the seminoma has spread beyond the lymph glands (this is rare) you would also be treated with 3 or 4 courses of chemotherapy.

Radiotherapy

46 Radiotherapy treats cancer by using high-energy rays which destroy the cancer cells, while doing as little harm as possible to the normal cells. It is often used to treat seminoma but not usually to treat teratoma.

Planning your treatment

47 To ensure that you receive maximum benefit from your radiotherapy it has to be carefully planned. On your first few visits to the radiotherapy department you will be asked to lie under a large machine called a simulator which takes X-rays of the area to be treated.

48 Treatment planning is a very important part of radiotherapy and it may take several visits before the radiotherapist (the doctor who plans your

treatment) is satisfied with the result.

49 Marks will be drawn on your skin to help the radiographer (who gives you your treatment) to position you accurately and to show the exact place for the rays to be directed. At the beginning of your treatment you will be given instructions on how to look after the skin in the area being treated. You will be told whether you can wash the marked areas of skin. Do not rub the area, as this may make it sore. Perfumed soaps, talcs, deodorants and lotions may also make your skin sore and should not be used.

50 Before radiotherapy is given, the radiographer will position you carefully on the couch and make sure you are comfortable. During your treatment, which only takes a few minutes, you will be left alone in the room but you will be able to talk to the radiographer who will be watching you carefully from an adjoining room. Radiotherapy is not painful but you do have to lie still for a few minutes while your treatment is given.

Side effects

51 Radiotherapy to the abdomen can cause side effects such as feelings of sickness (nausea), tiredness, and diarrhoea. Most of these side effects are mild and can be treated successfully with drugs. Anti-sickness tablets (anti-emetics) will usually be given to you at the start of radiotherapy. It is important to let your doctor know if you are having any problems. Any side effects should gradually disappear once your course of treatment is over.

52 While you are having radiotherapy it is important to drink plenty of fluids and have a healthy diet. If you don't feel like eating you could try supplementing your meals with high calorie drinks, which are available at most chemists (some are also available on prescription). During your treatment you should try to get as much rest as you can, especially if you have to travel a long way each day for treatment.

53 Radiotherapy does not make you radioactive and it is perfectly safe for you to be with other people, including children, throughout your treatment.

When is it given?

54 Radiotherapy is given to men with seminoma either to prevent the cancer

coming back after surgery or to treat disease that has spread to the glands at the back of the abdomen. It is a highly successful treatment, which will cure almost all men with this type of cancer.

55 The treatment is given in the hospital radiotherapy department usually as daily sessions from Monday to Friday, with a rest at the weekend. The length of your treatment will be decided by your doctor, but the whole course normally lasts from two to four weeks.

Chemotherapy

56 Chemotherapy is the use of anti-cancer (cytotoxic) drugs to destroy cancer cells. They work by disrupting the growth of cancer cells and as they circulate in the blood, they can reach cancer cells all over the body. The drugs most commonly used to treat testicular cancer are cisplatin, etoposide and bleomycin.

57 Chemotherapy may be given to men with teratoma, either to prevent the cancer coming back after surgery or to treat any cancer that has spread to the glands at the back of the abdomen, or elsewhere in the body. Men with seminoma usually have chemotherapy if there are a lot of cancer cells in the glands at the back of the abdomen, or if the seminoma has spread beyond the lymph glands.

58 Chemotherapy using a single dose of just one drug is also being tried to treat seminoma if the cancer does not seem to have spread. This is an alternative to radiotherapy to the glands at the back of the abdomen. Chemotherapy may also occasionally be used to shrink down a large testicular cancer before surgery so that it can be removed more easily.

59 The chemotherapy drugs are given by injection into a vein (intravenously). Chemotherapy is given as several courses of treatment which may last from two to five days, depending on the type of chemotherapy, followed by a rest period of a few weeks, which allows your body to recover from any side effects of the treatment. Chemotherapy for testicular cancer will usually mean spending a few days in hospital every three weeks from two to four times. If the cancer has spread to other parts of the body, four to six courses of chemotherapy may be necessary, or the treatment may be given weekly.

60 Treatment for testicular cancer is very successful, and the cancer does not usually come back after standard chemotherapy treatment.

High dose chemotherapy with stem cell support

61 High dose chemotherapy may be used if the standard chemotherapy does not completely get rid of the cancer cells (which is rare) or if the cancer is very advanced when it is found and there is a high risk that standard chemotherapy will not destroy all of the cancer cells.

62 This treatment involves giving very high doses of chemotherapy to try to destroy all the testicular cancer cells. As these high doses also damage cells in the bone marrow, certain cells in your blood called peripheral blood stem cells are collected and stored before treatment begins, then returned to the blood afterwards.

Side effects

63 While the chemotherapy drugs are acting on the cancer cells in your body they may also temporarily reduce the number of normal cells in your blood. When these cells are in short supply, you are more likely to get an infection and to tire easily. It is important to let your GP or cancer specialist know straight away if you feel unwell or develop a temperature at any time during your treatment. During chemotherapy your blood will be tested regularly and, if necessary, you will be given antibiotics to treat any infection. If the number of white blood cells drops below a certain level you may be given a drug known as a haematopoietic growth factor (GCSF) to stimulate the bone marrow.

64 Chemotherapy can cause changes in kidney function and your doctors will take regular blood tests to see how well your kidneys are working.

65 Some of the chemotherapy drugs can cause nausea and vomiting. This can be helped by taking anti-sickness drugs (anti-emetics) which your doctor can prescribe.

66 Some chemotherapy drugs can make your mouth sore and cause small ulcers. Regular mouthwashes are important and the nurse will show you how to use these properly.

67 If you don't feel like eating during treatment, you could try replacing some meals with nutritious drinks or a soft diet.

68 Hair loss is another common side effect. People who lose their hair often wear wigs, hats or scarves. You may be entitled to a free wig from the National Health Service. A doctor or the nurse looking after you will be able to arrange for a wig specialist to visit you. Your hair will grow back within 3–6 months.

69 One of the drugs (bleomycin) can occasionally cause inflammation in the lungs and this can lead to shortness of breath. This is usually mild, but if it becomes a problem your doctor may stop or change the drug.

70 Another drug (cisplatin) can cause tinnitus (ringing in the ears) and you may lose the ability to hear some high pitched sounds. This usually decreases when the treatment ends. You may also notice numbness or tingling in your hands and feet or difficulty doing up buttons. Your hands and feet may also become more sensitive to the cold. This is due to the effect of the drug on the nerves.

71 Although they may be hard to bear at the time, these side effects will usually disappear once your treatment is over.

72 Chemotherapy affects people in different ways. Some people find they are able to lead a fairly normal life during their treatment, but many find they become very tired and have to take things much more slowly. Just do as much as you feel like and try not to overdo it.

Follow up

73 After your treatment has been completed, your doctor will want you to have regular check-ups, blood tests, scans and X-rays. These will continue for several years. If you have any problems, or notice any new symptoms in between these times, you should let your doctor know as soon as possible.

Effect on sex life and fertility

74 One of the commonest questions asked by men before treatment for testicular cancer is whether their sex life will be affected. The important thing to remember is that the removal of one testicle will not affect your sexual performance or your ability to father children, if the other testicle is healthy. This is because the remaining healthy testicle will produce more testosterone and sperm to make up for the removal of the affected testicle.

75 Chemotherapy usually causes infertility during and for a time after treatment in men with testicular cancer. This is usually temporary but for some men it may be permanent. For this reason it is usually advisable to store sperm before starting chemotherapy treatment. The rate at which the sperm count recovers varies from person to person, but it generally returns to normal within two to three years.

76 The effect of chemotherapy on semen (the liquid that contains the sperm) and sperm is uncertain. Because of this it is advisable to use a condom during treatment and for about a month after treatment (this protects your partner and avoids any stinging sensation for your partner). Although there is no evidence that chemotherapy can harm children fathered after the treatment has finished, doctors usually advise that you avoid having a child for about a year after treatment.

77 Some men with testicular cancer have a low sperm count before they start any treatment, and sometimes successful treatment with chemotherapy may actually cause the sperm production to improve.

78 Sometimes it is necessary to surgically remove lymph glands in the abdomen, if they are still enlarged after radiotherapy or chemotherapy. Unfortunately, this can affect your fertility, as the operation can damage the nerves that control the discharge of sperm through the penis (ejaculation). However, new surgical techniques mean that this problem can usually be avoided. If there is a possibility that you may need such surgery, and if you are fit enough to produce sperm samples for storage before treatment starts, some of your sperm can be stored.

79 Although this further surgery may make it more difficult for you to father a child, it will have no physical effect on your ability to get an erection or have an orgasm.

80 Radiotherapy does not normally cause sterility. However, a small dose of radiation does reach the remaining testicle. There is no evidence that this radiotherapy has any effect on children fathered after the treatment, but men are usually advised to use contraceptives for

7

6–12 months after treatment has ended.

81 Any course of treatment may make you too tired to be interested in sex. This is called loss of libido and is common to many illnesses, not just cancer. It is worrying, but remember that it is a temporary side effect and once treatment is over and your body begins to return to normal, your libido will also return.

82 Sexual problems are very personal and very important and talking about them can be a great help. Although this can sometimes be difficult, once they have summoned up the courage to talk openly to their partners, many men find that their fears of rejection are unfounded. Sexual relationships are built on many things including love, trust and common experiences. You may even find a new closeness after talking through a problem with your partner.

83 In some cases, your doctor, nurse, close friend or relative may also be able to offer help and advice. Some hospitals have nurses or social workers who have been specially trained to help people with sexual problems.

84 One common fear is that cancer cells can be passed on to your partner during sex. This is not true. Cancer is not infectious and it is perfectly safe for you to have sexual intercourse.

Sperm storage before treatment

85 If your sperm is suitable and you would like to store some for the future, you will need to produce a number of sperm samples over a period of a few days. These can be frozen and stored for some time by the hospital. When you want to father a child, your sperm can be thawed and used to artificially inseminate your partner.

86 Unfortunately, not every man has sperm suitable for banking. To be successfully stored, it is thought that a sample must contain a certain number of active sperm cells, which would be able to fertilise a female egg. However, new techniques now make it possible for less active sperm to be effective.

87 It is best to discuss possible sperm storage with your doctor before your treatment starts, so that tests can be done to check your sperm count.

88 For many patients with cancer, the cancer unit will provide free sperm banking. But if the hospital has to pay for this service, they may need to charge the patient. The cost can vary between hospitals.

89 Sometimes your doctor may feel that it is important to start chemotherapy treatment quickly. In this situation there may not be enough time to arrange for sperm banking to be done before the treatment starts.

Your feelings

90 Most people feel overwhelmed when they are told they have cancer, even if the chance of cure is very high, as it usually is with testicular cancer. Many different emotions arise which can cause confusion and frequent changes of mood. You might not experience all the feelings associated with being diagnosed with testicular cancer, but they may occur. This does not mean, however, that you are not coping with your illness.

91 Reactions differ from one person to another – there is no right or wrong way to feel. These emotions are part of the process that many people go through in trying to come to terms with their illness. Partners, family members and friends often experience similar feelings and frequently need as much support and guidance in coping with their feelings as you do.

Questions

92 Concerns about the future – as well as about medical tests and treatments, hospital stays, and sexuality – are common. Talking with doctors, nurses, or other members of the health care team may help ease fear and confusion. Patients should ask questions about their disease and its treatment and take an active part in decisions about their medical care. Patients and family members often find it helpful to write down questions as they think of them to prepare for the next visit to the doctor. Taking notes during talks with the doctor can be a useful aid to memory. Patients should ask the doctor to repeat or explain anything that is not clear.

93 Most people want to know what kind of cancer they have, how it can be treated, and how successful the treatment is likely to be. The following are some questions patients might want to ask the doctor:

- I would like my partner/friend/family member to be with me during this consultation. Is that OK?
- What type of testicular cancer do I have?
- What tests are you going to do?
- Why – what are you looking for?
- After the tests will you know for sure whether I have cancer and if it has spread?
- Are they painful?
- How should I prepare?
- How long do the results take?
- Can you do a biopsy instead of removing my testicle?
- Can I have a fake testicle (prosthesis) put in during my operation?
- What are the blood tests for?
- What stage is my testicular cancer?
- How likely is it to be cured?
- Can it still be cured if it comes back after I am treated?
- Are there any treatment choices?
- Is it possible to keep working during treatment?
- How will you know if the treatment has worked?
- Am I likely to be able to father children after my treatment?
- Will the treatment affect my sex life?
- Should I have sperm banking before my treatment starts?
- Are there any clinical trials for testicular cancer treatment?
- How will you know if the cancer comes back?
- For how long will I need to come back for tests after my treatment has finished?
- Who can I talk to about problems with sex and fertility?
- Does the hospital offer counselling?
- How should I talk about the disease with my family and children?
- My son/brother is worried he might get testicular cancer. What should I tell him?

94 If you have testicular cancer there is further information that you might need – on new treatments, or individual drugs for example. Information is important when you have cancer and there are several organisations who can provide it and help with making choices. They produce ranges of literature, web sites and helplines to make it easier for you and your family to discuss concerns and gather more information.

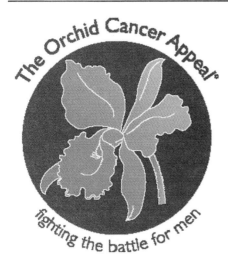

The Orchid Cancer Appeal

Formed in 1996 the Orchid Cancer Appeal was the first registered charity dedicated to funding research into diagnosis, prevention and treatment of both testicular and prostate cancer as well as promoting awareness of these previously-neglected diseases.

As well as funding cutting-edge research into men's cancers, the Orchid Cancer Appeal has produced a range of leaflets and other resource material free of charge to help people understand these cancers and their treatment.

If you would like more information on testicular or prostate cancer contact us.
Tel: 020 7601 7808
www.orchid-cancer.org.uk

7 Urethral cancer

Introduction

1 The urethra is the 'water-pipe' which runs through the penis and drains urine from the bladder to the outside world. Tumours of the urethra are very rare. Despite being much longer than its female equivalent, tumours occur here less often than in women.

Presenting features

2 Symptoms are usually those of difficulty in passing urine. Sometimes there is a bloody discharge from the penis or a painful lump. Sometimes abscesses develop which can discharge from the shaft of the penis. If there has been spread of the disease it may be possible to feel some lumps in the groin.

Risk factors

3 Long-standing inflammation of the urethra seems to be the biggest risk factor for developing the disease. It may occur as a result of repeated sexually transmitted diseases, infection with the human papilloma virus (HPV) or a narrowing (stricture) of the urethra. As many as three-quarters of those developing the disease will have had had a urethral stricture in the past. Most men who develop the disease are over 50 years old.

Diagnosis

4 Cystoscopy and biopsy of the urethra is the investigation of choice. It involves a telescopic camera being passed along the urethra so that the blockage or narrowing can be inspected and if necessary a piece of tissue taken for microscopic analysis. A urine specimen may be examined for abnormal cells (urine cytology). A CT scan (body scan) examines for any spread of the disease to the rest of the body.

Treatment

5 Treatment depends on how advanced the tumour is and whether or not it is found towards the tip or the base of the penis. Early tumours may be treated endoscopically (through the urethra) with a specially designed telescope called a cystoscope. Here the tumour can be cut away using a loop of wire through which electricity flows.

6 If the tumour is more extensive and invades deeper into the surrounding tissues then more extensive surgery is required. For tumours arising near the tip of the penis a partial amputation of the penis may be required to remove all the disease. For tumours arising nearer the base of the urethra then quite extensive and radical surgery may be required. For extensive disease, chemotherapy is now being used in combination with surgery with good results.

7

Notes

Chapter 8
Cruise control (endocrine system)

Contents

1 Breast cancer

Introduction

1 Yes, men can get breast cancer, though luckily it is very rare. Only about 1% of all breast cancers occur in men; it is commonest in men over 60. There is a small amount of breast tissue behind each nipple and it is here that the cancer can develop.

Causes

2 It is not possible to say with certainty what causes male breast cancer, but there are some factors which are known to increase the likelihood of it occurring. These include:

- Having close relatives (male or female) who have had breast cancer.
- Having close relatives who have had cancer of the ovary or colon.
- Exposure to repeated doses of radiation, especially when young.

3 If you think that you fall into one of the above categories, talk to your GP.

Symptoms

4 The usual symptom is a lump in the breast, or a change in its shape or size. Other symptoms include changes in the shape of the nipple, a discharge from the nipple and a rash on or around the nipple.

Diagnosis

5 An ultrasound scan is used to get a picture of the lump. A sample of cells from the lump will also be taken (by needle aspiration or needle biopsy) for

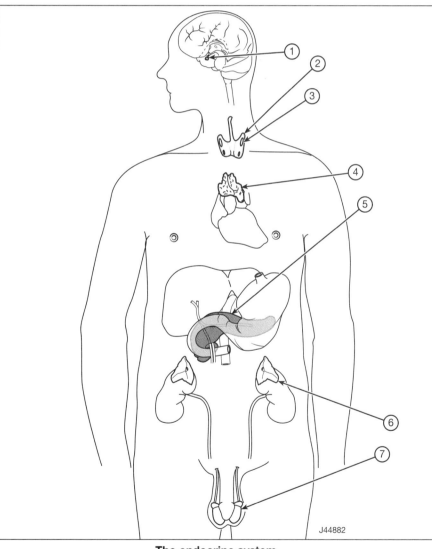

The endocrine system

1 *Pituitary gland*	4 *Thymus gland*	6 *Adrenal gland*
2 *Thyroid gland*	5 *Pancreas*	7 *Testes*
3 *Parathyroid gland*		

J44882

8

examination. These tests will show whether the lump is cancerous.

Treatment

6 Treatment for male and female breast cancer is essentially the same. One or more of the following may be used, depending on the type of cancer and how far it has spread:

- Surgery to remove the affected tissue, and maybe the lymph nodes in the armpit.
- Hormone therapy to reduce the level of oestrogen in the blood. Most breast cancers require oestrogen for their growth.
- Chemotherapy to destroy cancer cells which may be spreading elsewhere in the body.
- Radiotherapy to destroy the cancer cells, either in the original site or (if they have spread) elsewhere.

2 Pancreatic cancer

Introduction

1 The pancreas is a complex organ sitting in the loop of the duodenum (small intestine). It has a number of jobs, not least the controlling of blood sugar levels through the secretion of insulin from discrete 'islands' studded in the pancreas. The surrounding tissue is more concerned with producing digestive enzymes, particularly those for breaking down fat. It is in these parts of the pancreas that cancer is more likely to arise.

2 Although relatively rare it is unfortunately one of the most dangerous, with a poor survival rate, and is one of the 10 most common causes of cancer death in the UK. Men suffer from it twice as often as women and it is slightly higher in black men.

3 One of great problems for diagnosis is the lack of any symptoms until late in the development of the condition. There is also a difference in survival depending on where tumour arises in the pancreas.

Symptoms

4 These tend to develop over months rather than weeks and include:

- Pain in the upper abdomen under the rib cage which seems to go through to the back as well.
- Weight loss and lack of appetite.
- Jaundice and white motions which tend to float in the toilet can be a sign of later disease.

Diagnosis

5 MRI and CT scans are the most useful tools although endoscopy (a long flexible telescope) with the insertion of a small tube (stent) can help release any obstruction which may be causing jaundice. At the same time a small sample (biopsy) can be taken for further tests.

Treatment

6 Surgical removal is the only realistic chance of cure, but for most men it will be a matter of relieving the pain. Thankfully this is possible using pain killers and sometimes a nerve block.

Prevention

7 There are no hard and fast rules regarding prevention, although moderate alcohol consumption and a low fat diet may reduce your risk.

3 Cancer of the pituitary gland

Introduction

1 Often described as the 'body's orchestral conductor', the pituitary is a complex gland sitting at the base of the

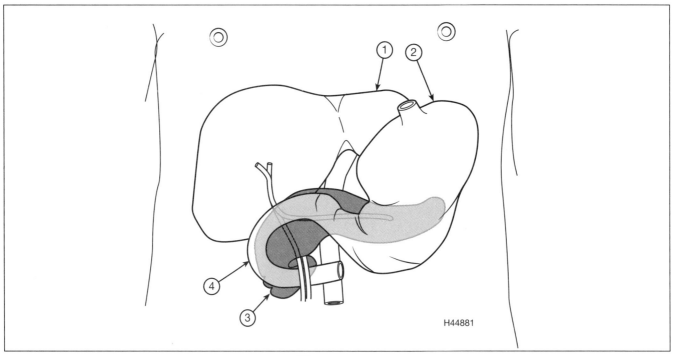

The pancreas

| 1 Liver | 2 Stomach | 3 Pancreas | 4 Duodenum |

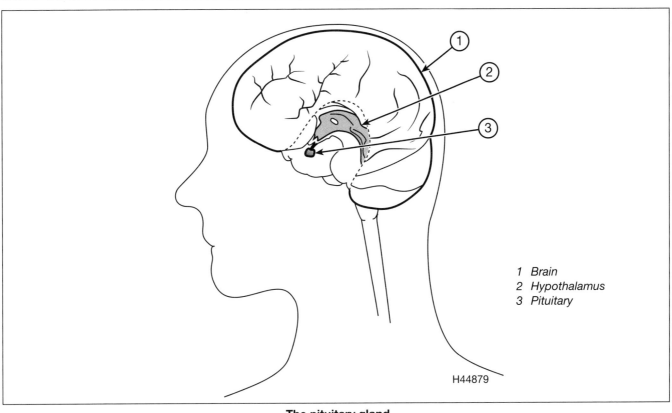

1 Brain
2 Hypothalamus
3 Pituitary

H44879

The pituitary gland

brain. It produces a number of hormones which collectively determine to a large extent the way the body functions. Cancer of this important part of the brain is fortunately rare and its treatment is increasingly successful.

2 The effect of the tumours will depend on whether or not they produce hormones which act on distant parts of the body. Most of these tumours are non-malignant, so spread from the gland is not a problem. Even so, the hormones they produce, or the pressure from the size of the tumour, can cause their own serious problems.

Symptoms

3 These will depend on the type of tumour, the hormone it is producing or preventing, and any pressure on surrounding tissues.

- Impotence can result from excess production of the hormone prolactin which suppresses testosterone production from the testes.
- Excess stimulation of the adrenal glands near the kidney can produce a condition called Cushing's Syndrome with characteristic 'moon

face' appearance and high blood pressure.
- Visual disturbances can occur from pressure on the optic nerves which run very close to the pituitary.
- Lack of stimulation of the thyroid gland in the neck can lead to hypothyroidism, with symptoms of lethargy, thick skin and weight gain.

Diagnosis

4 The warning signs for the doctor will come from what you describe as happening to you. The symptoms can arise gradually over a prolonged period of time so the penny doesn't always drop immediately. Blood tests for abnormally low or high levels of hormones can provide invaluable clues, but MRI or CT scans of the brain can often show the tumour. Although these tumours tend to be slow-growing, early diagnosis makes successful treatment all the more likely.

Treatment

5 A great deal depends on the type of tumour. Chemotherapy, radiotherapy and surgery are used often together and this may require hormone replacement

on a regular basis to make up for the loss of tissue that previously produced the essential hormones.

4 Cancer of the thyroid

Introduction

1 The thyroid gland sits in the throat just below the Adam's Apple (larynx). It has the job of regulating the body's metabolism. Too much thyroxine – its secreted hormone – makes the body work too fast, with the heart beating too quickly. Too little and the body is sluggish with a slow heart rate. A over- or under-active thyroid does not necessarily indicate the presence of cancerous cells.

2 Cancer of the thyroid is more common in women and previous exposure to radiation may be part of the cause. It is rare, one in 100 of all cancers are of the thyroid. It is more common in people over 40 years old. The good news is that successful treatment for thyroid cancer is amongst the highest for any cancers.

8

Symptoms

3 These depend on the type of thyroid cancer as they can arise in different parts of the gland. The majority tend to spread outside of the gland itself. Symptoms include:

- A painless lump in the throat.
- Difficulty or pain on swallowing.
- Hoarse voice.

Causes

4 There are no known causes of thyroid cancer other than the possible effect of direct radiation. Therefore there is little to advise on prevention. Thankfully it is a rare cancer.

Diagnosis

5 Examination of your neck and blood tests by your GP will provide most clues to the diagnosis but ultrasound, MRI or CT scanning can give definitive diagnosis particularly after a biopsy (taking a small sample of thyroid tissue).

Treatment

6 Surgical removal of the entire gland will often make survival possible. This can be done alongside radioactive iodine, which will only affect the thyroid gland or the metastases. As a result you will need thyroxine replacement, the normal hormone produced by the thyroid gland. Around 95% of people will survive their cancer.

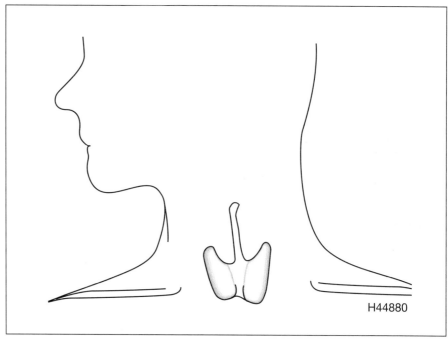

H44880

The thyroid gland

Chapter 9
Chassis and bodywork (bones and skin)

Contents

1 Bone metastases

Introduction

1 The process of metastasis is when cancer, which has developed in one area of the body, spreads and invades another area. Bone is a common site of metastasis for several types of cancers including: prostate, kidney, lung, breast and thyroid cancers, and multiple myeloma.

2 Cancerous cells, once present in the bone, can cause damage which gives rise to the uncomfortable symptoms often experienced by cancer patients with bone metastases. These bone complications are often referred to as skeletal related events (SREs). Bone metastases are treated by preventing SREs.

The bone

3 Bone is a type of connective tissue made up of minerals, such as calcium and phosphate, and the protein collagen. The outer layer of the bone is called the cortex and the spongy centre of the bone is called bone marrow. Bone tissue is porous and alive, with blood vessels running through it.

4 Like any other part of the body, the bone has to be broken down and replaced to keep its structural integrity. Healthy adult bone is continuously reshaped in response to stresses and strains (remodelled) through a process of bone resorbtion and bone formation. Two kinds of cells are involved in this process: osteoblasts (bone-forming cells) and osteoclasts (cells that break down, or resorb, bone).

5 Bones carry out a number of functions in the body:

- The skeleton provides structural support for the body.
- Bones store and release minerals that the body needs to function.
- Bone marrow produces and stores blood cells.

How does cancer spread to the bone?

6 When cancer cells break away from a cancerous tumour (a primary tumour), they can travel to other parts of the body through the bloodstream or the lymph vessels moving through the bloodstream or lymphatic system. Cancer cells can then lodge in an organ at a distant location and establish a new (secondary) tumour (see also *Brain cancer* in Chapter 5).

7 Secondary tumours that spread to bone (bone metastases) are not the same as primary bone cancer that starts in the bone (sarcoma). A tumour that has metastasised to bone is made up of abnormal cancer cells from the original tumour site and not of bone cells.

8 When cancer cells spread to the bone, they commonly lodge in the spine, rib cage, pelvis, limbs, and skull.

9 In cancer, the normal bone remodelling process is disturbed. Once cancerous cells are present in the bone, they cause abnormal 'dissolving' or wearing away of portions of the bone. This dissolving activity leaves holes called 'osteolytic lesions'. Bones are left fragile and weak so that they break or are prone to fracture.

9 In prostate cancer the tumour may stimulate bone to form and build up abnormally and the areas of bone resorbtion are therefore not filled. These areas of new bone are known as 'osteosclerotic lesions'. There is not the appropriate coupling between bone breakdown and bone formation, so the bone gets worn away and thinned. The result is fragile bone that can easily fracture or collapse.

What are the symptoms of bone metastases?

Bone pain

10 Pain is the most common symptom of bone metastases and is usually the first symptom that people notice. At first the pain may come and go and tends to be worse at night or with bed rest. Eventually the pain may increase and become severe. Obviously, not all pain indicates bone metastases. Your doctor can help distinguish between pain from metastases and aches and pains from other sources.

Fractures

11 Bone metastases can weaken bones, putting them at risk of fractures. In some cases, a fracture is the first sign of bone metastases. The long bones of the arms and legs and the bones of the spine are the most common sites of fracture.

9

Spinal cord compression

12 When cancer metastasises to the spine, it can squeeze the spinal cord. The pressure on the spinal cord may not only cause pain, it may cause numbness or weakness in the legs, problems with the bowels or bladder, or numbness in the abdominal area.

High blood calcium levels

13 High levels of calcium in the blood (hypercalcaemia) can be caused when calcium is released from the bones during the remodelling process. High calcium levels may cause nausea, thirst, constipation, tiredness, confusion and/or reduce your appetite, part of the reason for weight loss, another feature of cancer. If untreated, it may cause a coma or abnormal heart rhythm.

Other symptoms

14 If bone metastases affect the function of its bone marrow, other symptoms may be experienced depending on the type of blood cell affected. Red blood levels may drop, causing anaemia that leads to symptoms of tiredness, weakness, and shortness of breath. If white blood cells are affected, the person may develop infections that cause fevers, chills, fatigue or pain. If the number of platelets – a special cell involved in blood clotting - drops, abnormal bleeding may occur, a common first sign. It is usually noticed after brushing your teeth or by a small cut refusing to stop bleeding.

How are bone metastases diagnosed?

X-rays

15 Radiographic examination (X-rays) can provide information about what part of the skeleton the cancer has spread to, as well as the general size and shape of the tumour or tumours.

16 The damaged areas usually show up as dark spots on the X-ray film. But bone metastases often do not show up on X-rays unless the cancer is well-advanced.

Bone scan

17 Bone scans can detect bone metastases earlier than X-rays can. They also allow the doctor to monitor the health of all the bones in the body, including how they are responding to treatment.

18 In a bone scan, the person is given an injection of a low amount of radioactive material. The radioactive substance is attracted to diseased bone cells throughout the body. Diseased bone appears on the bone scan image as darker, dense areas.

Computerised tomography (CT) scan

19 The CT scan provides X-ray images to look at cross-sections of organs and bones in the body. Rather than provide one image as a conventional X-ray does, the CT scanner takes many pictures as it rotates around the body. A computer combines the images into one picture to show if cancer has spread to the bones. It is particularly helpful in showing osteolytic metastases that may be missed with the bone scan.

Magnetic resonance imaging (MRI)

20 MRI scans use radio waves and strong magnets instead of X-rays to provide pictures of bones and tissues. They are particularly useful in looking at the spine.

Laboratory tests

21 Bone metastases can cause a number of substances, such as calcium and alkaline phosphatase, to be released into the blood in amounts that are higher than normal. Blood tests for these substances can help diagnose bone metastases.

How can bone metastases be treated?

Introduction

22 The two main aims in the treatment of bone metastases are, firstly, to relieve the symptoms experienced by the patient and to ensure they are made more comfortable, and secondly, to reduce the number of cancer cells in the primary tumour and bone where possible.

23 There are several treatment options. Radiotherapy is an option used to relieve the symptoms of the disease, and chemotherapy or hormonal therapy are used either individually, or in combination to treat the underlying cancer. Bisphosphonates are drugs that inhibit bone destruction, reducing the incidence of skeletal complications and the need for radiotherapy treatment and surgery to bone.

Radiotherapy

24 Radiotherapy is the term used to describe the use of high-energy beams, often X-rays, to destroy cancer cells. An accelerator generates the beams, or alternatively, radioactive isotopes are used.

25 For bone metastases radiotherapy can be extremely effective at relieving pain and controlling the growth of tumour cells in the area of the bone metastases. It may also be used to prevent a fracture or as a treatment for spinal cord compression.

26 Typical radiotherapy treatment is administered once a day in 10 treatments over a two-week period, full effects of the treatment may take 2–3 weeks to occur. However, the reduction in bone pain may begin to occur between 7 and 10 days. During this time, patients are still advised to take painkillers prescribed by their doctor. This type of radiotherapy, which targets the area of bone affected, can cause some side effects. They include skin changes in the area being treated and a temporary increase in the symptoms of bone metastases.

Bisphosphonates

27 Bisphosphonates are drugs that restrict the action of the osteoclasts. They are not a treatment for the cancer itself but may help to reduce the breakdown of the bone and so reduce the risk of fracture and discomfort.

28 Several bisphosphonates are potent inhibitors of bone destruction (resorbtion) and are in clinical use for the treatment and prevention of osteoporosis, Paget's disease, hypercalcaemia caused by malignancy, tumour metastases in bone, and other bone ailments.

29 Intravenous (IV) bisphosphonates are the standard treatment for tumour-induced hypercalcaemia (TIH) and have become an integral part of the current treatment of skeletal metastases, reducing the incidence of skeletal complications and the need for radiotherapy treatment and surgery to bone. They are generally administered in the outpatient department or, where facilities allow, in the patient's own home or at the GP's surgery, once every 3–6 weeks. Some bisphosphonates can be taken by mouth as tablets but these

must be taken on an empty stomach an hour before food.

Radioisotopes

30 Radioisotopes are another method used to treat the symptoms experienced by patients with bone metastases. They are mildly radioactive substances (such as strontium-89) and are injected into a vein, usually in the arm. The radioisotope travels through the bloodstream to the bones, where it injures or destroys active cancer cells in the bone, relieving symptoms.

31 However, strontium-89 can temporarily reduce the number of normal red and white blood cells produced by the bone marrow. The reduction of white blood cells increases the risk of infection. The reduction in red blood cells may lead to anaemia, which can lead to the patient tiring easily. If the number of red cells is very low a blood transfusion may be necessary.

32 A swelling around the tumour area ('tumour flare') in the days following treatment may occur. Therefore, the patient may experience a temporary increase in pain.

Chemotherapy and hormone therapy

33 Chemotherapy drugs are used to kill cancer cells throughout the body. They may be taken orally or given intravenously.

34 Hormones are substances that occur naturally in the body and they control the activity and growth of normal cells. However in the cases of cancers such as prostate and breast, hormones can trigger the growth of those cancerous cells.

35 Hormonal therapy uses drugs to prevent hormones from forming or acting on cells to promote cancer growth. There are many different types of hormonal therapy and they all work in slightly different ways; in some cases several types of hormonal therapy may be given together. The therapy is administered either orally in the form of tablets or with injections.

36 Hot flushes and sweats are reported side effects. In most cases they are quite mild but on occasion some can be fairly severe.

37 The goals of chemotherapy and hormone therapy in patients with bone metastases are to control the tumour's growth, reduce pain, and reduce the risk of skeletal fractures.

Surgery

38 Very occasionally, when tests show that an area of bone is affected, the diseased bone is removed under anaesthetic and replaced with a pin or a replacement part. Tumours that have developed next to a joint such as the hip are also generally removed during an operation and then the joint is replaced.

Other therapies

39 Other treatments for bone metastases and their symptoms include physical therapy and drug and non-drug approaches to control pain. Many different drugs or combinations of drugs can be used to treat pain from bone metastases. Non-drug approaches to managing pain include the use of heat and cold, relaxation techniques and therapeutic beds or mattresses.

2 Malignant melanoma

Introduction

1 There are two main layers in the skin – the inner layer, the dermis, and the outer epidermis. The base of the epidermis is a single layer of active cells called the basal layer. This layer buds off new cells that are then pushed towards the surface, becoming flatter and harder

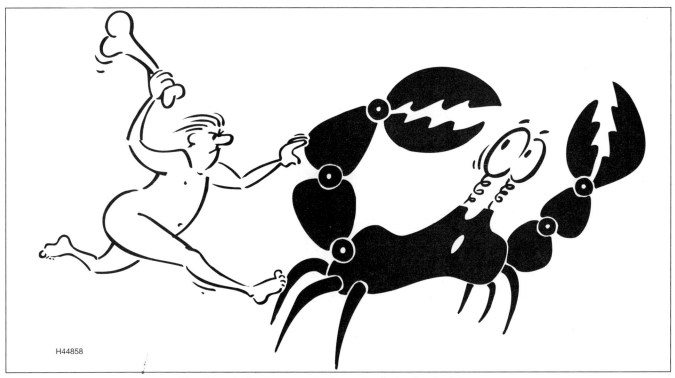

H44858

Treatments for bone metastases include physical therapy

9

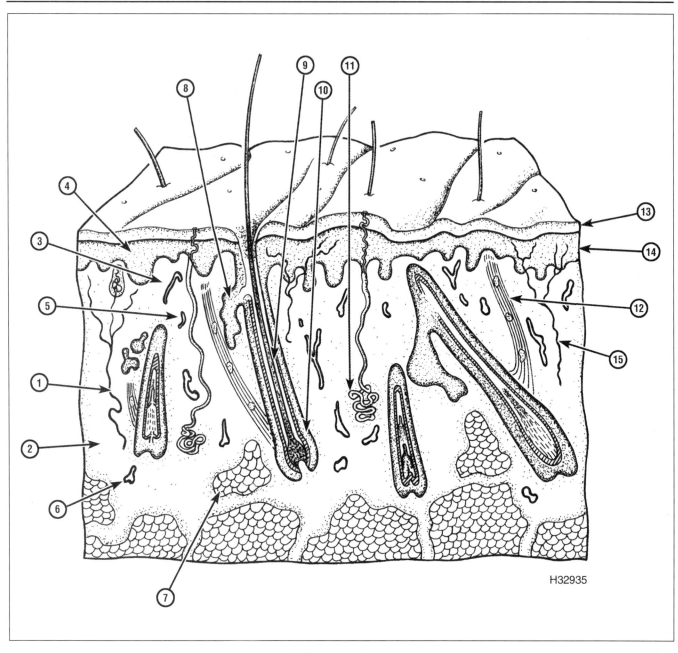

H32935

Skin components

1 Nerve	6 Blood vessel	11 Sweat gland
2 Subcutaneous tissue	7 Fat	12 Muscle
3 Papillary layer	8 Sebaceous (sweat) gland	13 Epidermis
4 Stratum corneum	9 Hair root	14 Dermis
5 Reticular layer	10 Hair bulb	15 Connective tissue

as they move outwards. This is the 'wear and tear' layer of the skin, and the cells on the surface are cast off. Some of the cells in the basal layer of the epidermis are called melanocytes. These cells contain a brown colouring matter (pigment) called melanin that is responsible for colouring the skin. A melanoma is a tumour that starts in one of these cells.

2 Malignant melanoma is still comparatively rare and has an incidence of 5 to 10 per 100,000 of the white population per year. The tumour is even less common in children. Only about two per cent of all malignant melanomas occur in people under 20 and only 0.3 to 0.4 per cent of them occur in children below puberty. The incidence in white people is 10 to 20 times greater than in black and dark-skinned peoples.

In the last 25 years, the incidence of malignant melanoma has increased more rapidly than that of any other tumour. The increases are greatest in adolescents and young adults. By far the most likely explanation of this is the increasing affluence in the Western world, and the sun-tan culture, that have led to a marked increase in skin exposure to sunlight.

3 About one cancer in 100 is a malignant melanoma. The incidence of this disease has doubled every ten years for the past 40 years. In children, melanoma may be present at birth (congenital) or may develop in infancy. In older children it is more likely to occur in skin that has been damaged by the sun. Certain other unusual conditions make melanoma more likely in children.

4 About half of malignant melanomas arise from pre-existing moles. Nearly everyone has pigmented moles, but only one in a million becomes malignant. Hairy moles hardly ever turn into malignant melanomas. Once you are suspicious of changes in a coloured skin mole, don't delay in reporting the condition for an expert opinion.

Symptoms

5 In white people, malignant melanomas occur most often on the upper part of the back in both men and women. In women, it is also equally common on the legs between the ankle and the knee. In black people, melanomas are very rare but when they do occur they are usually on the palms, soles and behind the finger and toe nails.

6 The signs of malignant change in a mole are very important to know. They are:

a) A change in shape, especially an increasingly irregular outline.

b) A change in size.

c) Increased projection beyond the surface.

d) A change in colour, especially sudden darkening and the development of colour irregularities appearing as different shades of brown, grey, pink, red or blue.

e) Itching or pain.

f) Softening or crumbling.

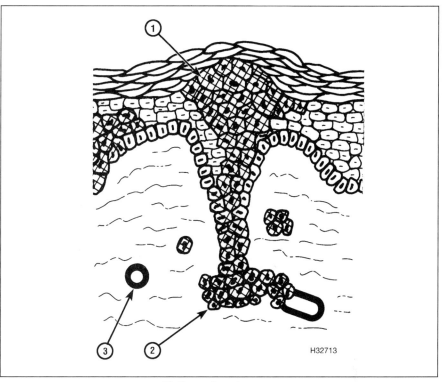

Malignant melanoma

1 Cancer cells in epidermis   2 Cancer cells spreading into dermis   3 Blood vessel

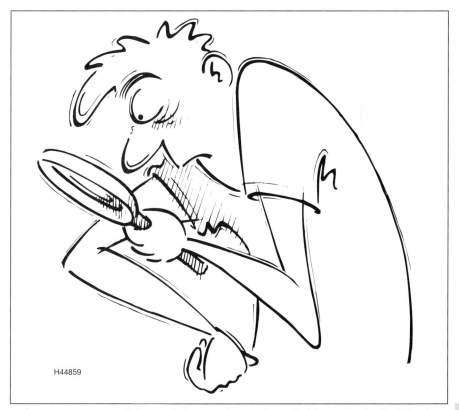

Once you are suspicious of changes in a coloured skin mole, don't delay in reporting the condition for an expert opinion

9

g) *The development of new satellite moles around the original one.*

h) *The development of a light or dark halo or ring around the mole.*

7 Report any of these changes to your doctor as a matter of urgency.

Causes

8 Melanomas are most common on areas exposed to the sun, but may occur anywhere on the skin. There is a definite link between sunbathing and the incidence of malignant melanomas. Probably the most dangerous type of sunbathing is a short, sharp period of intense exposure, either in a single day or over a short period such as a holiday.

9 Some white people are more likely to get melanomas than others. People with freckles, those with 20 or more birthmarks, and those who have had 3 or more severe sunburns, are at least 200 times more likely to get a melanoma than those with none of these features.

Diagnosis

10 There is only one way to make a positive and sure diagnosis of a malignant melanoma, or to exclude that diagnosis – to have a total biopsy of the suspected tumour. Margins of normal skin should be left all round. In this way the whole specimen is available for examination.

Prevention

11 Avoid deliberate and unnecessary prolonged exposure to the sun. Always cover up. Particular risk factors for melanoma are fair skin and inappropriate exposure to the sun with burning. White skin in childhood may be especially susceptible. Every precaution must be taken to protect the skin against the dangers of ultraviolet radiation.

12 T-shirts or other protective clothing should be worn during swimming. Effective sunscreen creams should be used, and it is best to stay indoors during the midday period when the ambient rays pass through the thinnest atmospheric distance and are thus most intense. Use sunscreen creams but don't rely on them to protect you entirely. It is better to avoid the direct rays of the sun by wearing a shirt.

Treatment

13 Melanomas are removed along with a wide area of normal-seeming tissue around them. A skin flap may be needed to cover the defect. In cases of treated melanomas with a thickness of 1 mm or less, the survival rate is 90 per cent. More than this and the outlook gets worse. This emphasises the importance of avoiding delay in reporting any suspicious changes.

3 Multiple myeloma

Introduction

1 Multiple myeloma is a cancer of the cells that produce antibodies, called plasma cells. It actually forms in more than one part of the active bone marrow of various bones. These are the regions in the body where blood cells are produced. Antibodies are proteins which attach themselves to bacteria, viruses or sometimes cancer cells. This helps the immune system to destroy them and so protect the body from infection and cancer.

2 For some reason the abnormal myeloma cells stop making useful antibodies and instead produce large quantities of a useless substance called Bence Jones protein. This has implications for more than simply the immune system, as the large amount of protein produced can block the fine tubes inside the kidneys.

3 Around one person in 30,000 will develop multiple myeloma, the majority being over the age of 50 years.

Symptoms

4 Like some other cancers, myeloma tumour can erode normal bone causing pain and fractures. This bone destruction

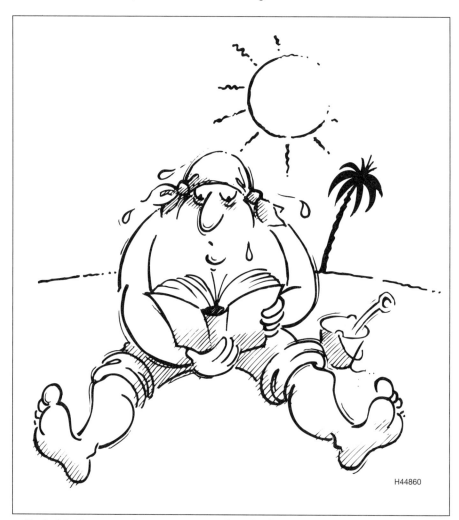

H44860

Probably the most dangerous type of sunbathing is a short, sharp period of intense exposure

can lead to high levels of calcium in the blood causing nausea, vomiting, loss of appetite, constipation, dehydration, drowsiness and confusion.

5 Normal blood cell production is crowded out so anaemia (lack of red blood cells) is often a feature with pallor, weakness, breathlessness on effort and fatigue. The reduction in production of normal antibodies results in increased liability to infection.

Causes

6 There may be a genetic element as the disease does seem to run to some extent in families, but it is also commoner after exposure to large doses of radiation.

Diagnosis

7 Obvious changes in the bones, most easily seen in the skull, may be visible on X-ray examination. However, the most effective test is to check the blood for anaemia and raised calcium and protein levels. The urine may contain large amounts of Bence Jones protein. One of the oldest tests was to gently heat a sample of urine to show a white jelly like protein appear in a similar way to egg white turning solid.

Treatment

8 Anaemia and infections can be treated with blood transfusions and antibiotics. Bone pain can be relieved by radiotherapy and pain-killers mixed with anti-inflammatory drugs. Chemotherapy can significantly prolong life but is aimed really at improving the quality of remaining life. Major progress has come from the use of bisphosphonates (see Section 1 of this Chapter).

---

4 Skin cancer

See that big round yellow thing hanging in the sky? It causes more cancer in the UK than anything else you can shake a pair of sunglasses at.
Don't be a mad dog, get out of the midday sun!

---

1 Not a lot of people know this:
- Skin cancer is the most common cancer in the UK, and not just in women.
- Your risk of growing an extra, unwanted, outside cancerous lump by the age of 74 is one in six.
- Even cloudy days can deliver 9/10ths of the dangerous UV rays.
- Some football shirts are so thin they let almost all the sun's UV radiation shine right through.
- Once the sunburn fades from this year's trip to Majorca it doesn't mean you're in the clear. Damage builds up under the skin just like rust under bodywork paint and can come back to haunt you in later years.
- Virtually all the risk comes from the sun and sun-beds… So cover up and close up!

Shades of the truth

- Use high factor sun-screens (30+ in sunnier climates). Slap loads on BEFORE you head into the sun and re-apply every 2 hours.
- Cover up, always; and that means when working or holidaying at home too.
- Get ahead and get a hat, a big hat.
- Get out of the midday sun when possible or else look for a nice bit of shade to relax or work in.
- Get those shades on to protect your (next) best assets!

2 All men, no matter what colour their skin, need to be sun-smart, but the guys with the following need to be extra careful even when working or playing outside in the UK, as well as abroad:
- Pale or freckled skin that doesn't tan or burns before it tans.

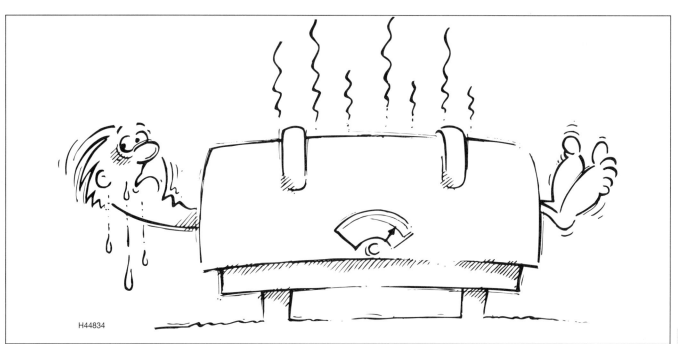

H44834

Virtually all the risk comes from the sun and sun-beds… So cover up and close up!

- Naturally red or fair hair and blue, green or grey eyes.
- A large number of moles (50 or more).
- Easy burnt skin, a history of sunburn or already had skin cancer.

Sunscreens and smokescreens

3 People get confused over sunscreens and can damage their skin through a false sense of security, remember:

- The higher the Sun Protection Factor (SPF) number, the greater the protection provided. A SPF above 15 gives high protection.
- Wearing sunscreen does not mean that you can stay out in the sun longer than recommended – it offers some protection, but should be used with cover-up clothing.
- It is very important to apply sunscreen thickly and evenly. Most people get a lot less protection than they think because they do not put enough sunscreen on their skin.
- Those parts of the body that are not usually exposed to the sun will tend to burn more easily. But also take extra care of ears, neck, bald patches, hands and feet.

Sun sense

4 The sun damages your bodywork by its Ultraviolet Radiation (UV) and there are two types:

UVA

- Results in early ageing and skin cancer.

UVB

- Most harmful, causes burning and skin cancer.

5 Tanned skin is damaged skin. It's a sign that damaged skin is trying to protect itself from the sun's ultraviolet rays. Even when you have a suntan, you can still get sunburn.

6 There are two main types of skin cancer.

Non-melanoma skin cancer

7 Most common form, often seen on the ear tips, nose, forehead and cheeks but is very curable.

8 Look out for:

- A new growth or sore that does not heal within four weeks.
- A spot or sore that continues to itch, hurt, crust, scab or bleed.

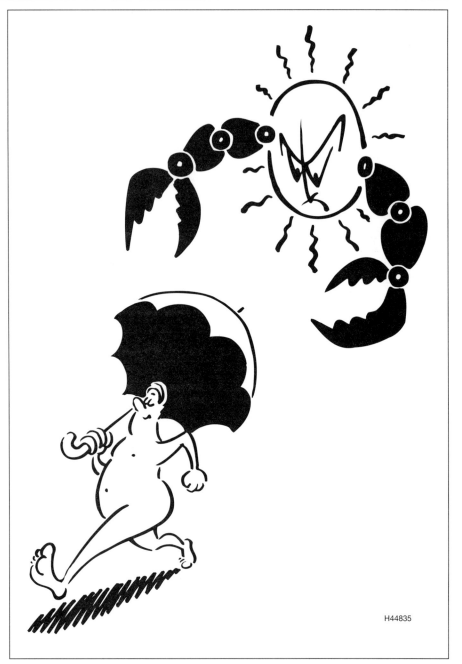

All men, no matter what colour their skin, need to be sun-smart

- Constant skin ulcers that are not explained by other causes.

Malignant melanoma

9 Most serious form and although relatively rare it is on the increase, especially in men. It most often appears as a changing mole or freckle but the good news is that early diagnosis is likely to produce a cure.

10 Mole maintenance, watch out for changes such as:

- Size.
- Colour.
- Shape.
- Itchiness.
- Bleeding.

11 Many skin changes will be harmless, but if you notice anything unusual, you should visit your doctor.

Reference

Contents

Grieving and coping with bereavement

Death is inevitably upsetting and may occur at any age, even in childhood. As we grow older, our contact with personal loss increases, but it may never get any easier to deal with.

Death in old age

The loss of an elderly relative or friend is supposed to be less painful. People will attempt to console you with well-intended comments such as, "Well, she had a good innings". Heads will nod, but a long innings often gives more reason to hope that death will never come.

Scale of misery

Psychologists often refer to a scale that rates life events in terms of the stress they can cause. The death of a spouse or child comes at the very top.

Predictable response

The scale is useful because it helps to demonstrate how you may feel when you have lost a loved one. The stages of the "grieving reaction" are listed below. While the order of these stages remains the same for almost everyone, the severity and duration of each will vary from person to person.

Denial
- "It can't be true. There's been some mistake."

Anger
- "It must be the doctor's fault. Why did they leave me?"

Guilt
- The next emotion, self-guilt, can be the most destructive. "How could I be so idiotic? It's all my fault." People will find the most unlikely things with which to whip themselves unmercifully. This stage can last a long time even when people rationalise the cause of their misery.

Acceptance
- After a variable amount of time there comes a period of acceptance. There is no fixed time for this period, which can even depend upon the community. People generally will profess to have come to terms with their loss before they have actually done so.

Coming to Terms
- Well-meaning folk will tell you that you'll get over it. The truth is that you never "get over" a major life event. What happens is that you come to terms with it; the pain diminishes gradually with time. It is not a smooth progression, however, and anniversaries, returning to places, or even casual mention of the person or some object or event will release waves of heartache.

Just to help me sleep

People close to the recently bereaved can be so shocked by the effect on their loved one that they may ask for, or even demand, sedatives from the doctor.

Indeed, this used to be the norm, and there can be no doubt that drugs will numb the pain of grief. Unfortunately, grief will not be denied; and if it is not allowed to take its course with the support of friends and relatives, it will resurface after the drugs and the support have gone.

People in grief then find themselves alone but with the heartache they should have had when help was at hand. People often talk of such an experience as "floating above the events" only to come down with a thump later on.

Effects underestimated

Most people underestimate the effects of bereavement on a person, until it happens to themselves. Some effects can be so bad that the bereaved person often will not realise that loss of interest in job or family, constant pacing of the floor, spontaneous weeping or complete loss of appetite are all normal and common manifestations of grieving. People close to the bereaved person may also become impatient as time wears on, again underestimating the extent of the effects of grief and the length of time they can be felt. It is at this point that true friends are worth their weight in gold. To know when to leave the person alone and when to sit and listen, often to the same story over and over again without interruption, is a gift that few people have nowadays. Bereavement can even affect the memory, and people will say they experienced a "complete blank" for a period following the death. Almost every facet of life can be and is affected – only the scale and duration varies between people.

Thankfully, there are professional agencies specialising in bereavement counselling which can be contacted through your GP. Nobody pretends that strangers are as good as friends or relatives, but they can often help people who have difficulty coming to terms with their loss.

Points to remember:
- People have different ways of expressing grief; there is no "normal way".
- Talk about it, even if it hurts.
- Don't be afraid to seek support from friends, relatives or your doctor.
- Aggression is natural, even towards close relatives and well-meaning neighbours. Doctors are a common focus of anger.
- Allow yourself time to grieve, and avoid drugs.

Support for those left behind, and love for those about to die, can help make life better for us all.

Getting the best from your GP and Pharmacist

Pharmacists are a great source of information. You can often see them quicker than your GP and many have a confidential area. They can advise whether you should see your GP.

Find a GP who suits you

The local library keeps a list of GPs in the area, as do the social services, but asking your mates can point you towards your kind of doctor.

Write down your symptoms before you see your doctor

It is easy to forget the most important things during the examination. Doctors home-in on important clues. When did it start? How did it feel? Did anyone else suffer as well? Did this ever happen before? What have you done about it so far? Are you on any medicines at present?

Arrive informed

Check out the internet for information before you go to the surgery. There are thousands of sites on health, men's health and cancer, but many of them are of little real use, so click on ones that are from recognised institutions or recommended ones such as malehealth.co.uk or NHS Direct online for up-to-date, accurate and unbiased information (see *Contacts*).

Ask questions

If a mechanic stuck his head under the bonnet of your car you would most certainly want to know what he intended doing. The doctor is about to lift the bonnet on your body – don't be afraid to ask why and what he is doing.

Don't beat about the bush

If you have a lump on your testicles say so. With a limited amount of consultation time there is otherwise a real danger of coming out with a prescription for a sore nose.

Listen to what they say

If you don't understand, say so. It helps if they write down the important points. Most people pick up less than half of what their doctor has told them.

If you want a second opinion say so

Ask for a consultant appointment by all means, but remember you are dealing with a person with feelings and not a computer. Compliment them for their attention first, then explain your anxiety.

Trust your doctor

But remember, there is a difference between trust and blind faith. Your health is a partnership between you and your doctor where you are the majority stakeholder.

Don't be afraid to ask to see your notes

Most doctors now show their patients what they are writing. Unfortunately, doctor's language can be difficult to understand. Latin and Greek are still in use although on the decline. Doctors use abbreviations in your notes so ask for explanations. Eg: *TATT* Tired all the time, *DNA* Did not attend, *FU2* You insulted him.

Expert Patients Programme

The Expert Patients Programme aims to help people live with long term conditions, maintain their health and improve their quality of life through lay led self management courses. People learn to regain as much control over their physical and emotional well-being as possible. It complements existing health care programmes and treatments, enabling patients to become more informed and better able to work in partnership with their doctor.

It is a generic, time-limited course, suitable for people who have any long-term conditions. It enables people to have greater confidence in dealing with their illness, experience less pain and fatigue, depression and anxiety.

To find out where your nearest Expert Patient Programme is being held please call or find out more from the website (see Contacts).

NHS Cancer Screening Programmes

The NHS Cancer Screening Programmes comprises two nationally co-ordinated screening programmes for breast and cervical cancer, the English Bowel Screening Pilot and Prostate Cancer Risk Management. The programme operates on the principle of Informed Choice, providing men and women with clear and balanced information from which they can make informed decisions about their health. Prostate Cancer Risk Management provides resources to enable men considering a prostate specific antigen (PSA) test to be given information concerning the benefits, limitation and risks associated with receiving a test, while the English Bowel Screening Pilot is evaluating the practicalities involved in implementing a national screening programme.

English Bowel Screening Pilot

Why screen for bowel cancer?

Bowel cancer is a major public health problem. It is the second most common cause of cancer deaths in the United Kingdom. At the moment research suggests that screening for bowel cancer could reduce deaths from the disease by 15 per cent. By finding and treating it early, a national screening programme for bowel cancer could save around 1200[1] lives each year.

What is bowel screening?

Screening involves looking for signs of disease in people who have no obvious symptoms. The aim is to find disease at an early stage when there is a better chance of it being successfully treated. If early signs of bowel cancer are found and the disease treated, not only can a life be saved, but also treatment can be less drastic.

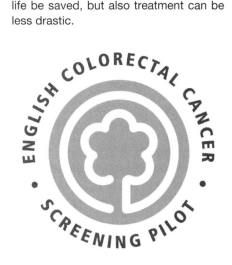

The English bowel screening pilot

The *National Screening Committee* (NSC) reviewed the evidence on bowel cancer screening and found that population screening of people over the age of 50 for non-visible (occult) blood in the faeces can reduce the death rate for bowel cancer[2]. The NSC recommended to Ministers that a pilot screening project be organised.

As a result of this recommendation, the *NHS Cancer Screening Programmes* established a pilot in 1999 in Coventry and Warwickshire. Over a two year period, both men and women aged between 50 and 69 who were registered with a participating GP were offered a Faecal Occult Blood test (FOBt) to complete at home and return to the lab for analysis.

The second stage of the pilot is now underway. Again men and women aged between 50 and 69 and registered with a participating GP based in Coventry, Rugby or North Warwickshire will automatically receive an invitation and offered a FOBt.

What is the test?

There are a number of ways of screening for bowel cancer. At the moment, the tests being considered are the FOBt (looking for blood in the stools) and Flexible Sigmoidoscopy (using a tube to look inside the lower part of the bowel). Research is still being conducted into the potential value of these tests and the possibility of them being used within a national screening programme.

The FOBt is the method that is currently being piloted in Rugby, Coventry and North Warwickshire. It is a simple test that can be completed at home. It is used to detect tiny amounts of blood in a sample of bowel motion. Individuals are asked to smear small samples from their bowel motion onto a special card supplied for this purpose. The test then needs to be sealed in a specially designed prepaid envelope and posted via Royal Mail to the screening laboratory for analysis. The obvious advantage of this test is that individuals can complete it in the privacy of their own home and so it may save some embarrassment.

What happens if the result is abnormal?

Approximately two out of every 100 people who complete a FOBt will have an abnormal result. Those who do will be offered further investigations, usually a colonoscopy (where a long flexible tube is used to look inside all of the bowel).

An abnormal result does not mean that an individual has cancer. It could be caused by a number of things, including what someone eats prior to the test; for example, recent consumption of red meat can affect the result. The test is an indication that something might be wrong, and not a diagnosis. For about 80 per cent of people, further investigation reveals that they do not have bowel cancer.

Are there any risks?

There are no risks associated with completing a FOBt. However tests used for further investigation do carry some risks. Such tests might include a colonoscopy or a barium enema which uses a special liquid to show up any abnormal areas on X-ray. Any risks are explained fully so that an informed choice on whether to proceed or not can be made before undergoing any further investigation.

Reasons for men not participating

The bowel screening pilot revealed that men are less likely to take an FOBt than women. There are a number of reasons for this, one being that some men perceive bowel cancer to be more serious, both in physical and psychosocial terms. They believe it could lead to pain and sickness and limit their social and personal relationships, as well as threatening their financial security. Because of this, men may avoid taking a FOBt through fear of a positive result.

The pilot also identified a number of other barriers to men completing a FOBt, including:

- Feeling an invasion of privacy.
- Embarrassment or discomfort talking about their bowels.
- Disgust at the procedure.
- Perceiving the process to be unhygienic.
- Work or other commitments not allowing time.
- Believing they are not at risk of bowel cancer and so do not need to complete a FOB test. This may be denial at getting older and so at higher risk.

When will screening be available nationally?

The second round of screening is currently taking place in Rugby, Coventry and North Warwickshire as part of the English bowel cancer screening pilot. The aim of the pilot is to find out as much as possible about the practicalities of introducing a national screening programme for bowel cancer.

Due to the success of the pilot the Government has announced its commitment to introducing a national bowel cancer screening programme and is currently developing plans to do so. However, it will take a number of years to put in place.

Who will be screened?

Medical evidence shows that the occurrence of bowel cancer increases with age, particularly over the age of 50. The typical bowel cancer patient is in their seventies, so it is important that screening takes place before that age. The Government has reaffirmed its commitment to introducing bowel cancer screening for the population most likely to benefit.

References

[1] Atkins, W. Implementing screening for colorectal cancer. *BMJ* 1999; 319:1212*3

[2] Hardcastle JD, Chamberlain JO, Robinson MHE, et al. Randomised controlled trial of faecal-occult-blood screening for colorectal cancer. *Lancet*, 1996;348:1472-147

The PSA test and screening for prostate cancer

The PSA test is a blood test, available from your GP. It helps doctors diagnose and manage prostate problems when a man has urinary symptoms and goes to his GP for diagnosis and treatment. The PSA blood test can indicate the presence of a prostate problem, which may sometimes turn out to be prostate cancer. The PSA test should not be referred to as 'the test for prostate cancer' as only rarely is it diagnostic of cancer. If PSA levels are raised, prostate biopsy will usually be necessary to reach a diagnosis.

Some people, including some doctors, are keen on using the PSA test to screen well men regularly for prostate cancer. A 'screening' system means that men, otherwise well and symptom free, over the age of about 45, receive regular invitations to visit their GPs for the PSA blood test which might indicate the need for further tests for prostate cancer.

The value of the PSA test for screening is the source of major global medical debate.

Current scientific evidence that PSA tests save men's lives from prostate cancer is equivocal. Whilst it seems obvious that it *should* save lives, clear evidence that it *does* save lives does not, as yet, exist. Many men with prostate cancer believe that their lives *were* saved because they had a PSA test, and are keen that all men have PSA tests regularly through a Screening Programme. Some specialists are also keen on the PSA test to screen for prostate cancer. Many other medical scientists and urological specialists have reservations about the usefulness of PSA as a potential screening test for prostate cancer in men without symptoms.

This is not just a UK puzzle. It is a global debate. No country has a routine population Screening Programme with the PSA test, except Luxembourg. The US does not, though the PSA test is used more commonly there than it is here. There are research studies going on in Europe to test the effectiveness of PSA screening in saving lives from prostate cancer. The results are not expected for several years yet.

The PSA test will not help identity all prostate cancers, and not all cancers it will help identify will need treatment. The aggressive prostate cancers which cause most concern, will not necessarily be picked by screening with the PSA test, as they can develop in the intervals between 'screening'.

Currently, there is no Screening Programme for prostate cancer in the UK. There is unlikely to be one unless there is a shift in the evidence or better screening tests become available.

Men with concerns about prostate cancer who have heard of the PSA test but have no symptoms can talk to their GP about it. Information about the PSA test is available under the NHS's Prostate Cancer Risk Management Programme. If a man still wants a PSA test after the consultation and consideration of the details, he can have one free on the NHS.

There is a difference between what is

'appropriate' to offer to a population and the choices an individual may wish to exercise for himself. Men should have the chance to weigh up the decision to pursue a PSA test for themselves. All men are individuals with different priorities, responsibilities, family background, medical histories, ages, and attitudes to risk. No 'one size' decision will fit all.

Making the PSA test available to men within a routine Screening Programme implies it is effective in saving lives. It also implies that taking part in a Screening Programme would definitely benefit the vast majority of men. Using the PSA test in the same way as cervical smears implies that the PSA test is similarly effective. We all wish it was so, but the evidence for this level of certainty does not yet exist. Using the PSA test in a Screening Programme would obscure disclosure of the uncertainties about the test, and the variable nature of prostate cancer. Being offered a PSA test through a Screening Programme could distract most men from asking appropriate questions about the test, and the cancer, and encourage them to assume that only benefits can arise from taking part, and that the risks are minor.

There are risks associated with being screened for prostate cancer. Many men would undergo treatment for prostate cancer detected as a result of the PSA test. Had they never been screened, the cancer itself may never have caused significant pain, discomfort or symptoms in their lifetime. The treatments for the condition are not without side effects. The ones which cause most concern are urinary incontinence and impotence. Thus the side effects of treatment could be worse than the cancer would have been. There is also an ethical problem. There is a risk of causing psychological distress by setting out to diagnose a cancer for which choosing no treatment is a viable option.

The PSA test is not without merit. Some men may be alerted to a potentially life-threatening condition and should not be prevented from having the opportunity of a PSA test. However, whilst some men may be alerted to a life-threatening condition many others will experience the side effects of treatment for a condition which, had they remained unaware of it, would never have caused them any major problems. It is impossible, at present, for medical science to tell an individual man with confidence which category he will fall into.

Many men will find it difficult to reconcile the uncertainty about the PSA test with decisions 'for' or 'against' having one. However, men are not helped to make an informed choice if the level of uncertainly and lack of clarity is minimised because it would be more 'comfortable'. Men cannot make an informed choice if they misunderstand the issues as clear and their attention is not drawn to the uncertain background of the PSA test when used as a screening test.

On the other hand, the active engagement of men with their own health needs is not supported by suppressing information about the PSA test, which is why men need to know about the PSA test and what it could mean for them.

Screening well men for prostate cancer will come in when an effective screening technology is developed, or when robust research evidence shows that men's lives are saved by the current test.

Scientists, doctors, policy makers and some patient groups continue to argue about the benefits of prostate cancer screening using the PSA test. Even if a Screening Programme is introduced, based on the PSA test or any other more effective test, decisions about screening should be made by each man himself.

Living with cancer

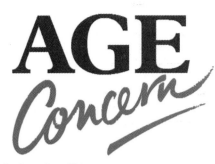

Introduction

People are living much longer than they used to. The longer we live the longer our bodies are exposed to cancer-causing chemicals and environmental factors (such as sunlight) which increase the risk of abnormal cells developing. As we age, our immune system also becomes less effective at identifying these abnormal cells and destroying them before they have a chance to develop into cancers. So most types of cancer are more common in older people.

- Cancer is twice as common in older men as women.
- 60-70% of all cancers now occur in people over 65.
- Lung cancer is the commonest serious cancer in people under 85.
- Prostate cancer is the commonest cancer in men over 85.
- A quarter of cancers of the stomach occur in people over 80.
- Prostate cancer is 22 times more common in older men than in younger men.
- 95% of a type of skin cancer (squamous cell carcinoma) occur in older people.

As we grow older we are more likely to suffer form a variety of aches and pains and other symptoms. It is easy to assume that new symptoms are just part of the ageing process and ignore them. However, any new symptoms should be discussed with your doctor so that he or she can decide whether they really are a normal part of the ageing process or not.

Prevention

Experts have estimated that more than 80% of cancers may be avoidable through changes that can be made to lifestyle and in the environment. Smoking and poor diet are believed to each account for one-third of all cancers. Most people know that healthy ageing includes trying to:

- Keep physically active.
- Eat a healthy diet.
- Keep your weight within the normal range.
- Give up smoking.
- Drink sensibly.

A diet rich in fruit and vegetables appears to protect against cancer of the stomach, oesophagus, large bowel and lung. This may be because of the vitamins and fibre they contain. Most people in the UK eat around three portions of fruit and vegetables a day rather than the 'five-a-day' that is recommended. (The 'five-a-day' logo has been developed by the Government to try and encourage greater consumption of fruit and vegetables.

There is also some evidence that by eating plenty of starchy and fibre-rich foods we may be helping to protect ourselves against bowel cancer. There may be a link between obesity and cancer of the prostate.

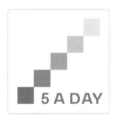

5 A DAY

Just Eat More
(fruit & veg)

Most common types of cancer in men

Lung Cancer

Lung cancer is a disease of middle and older age and most cases are detected after the age of 50. It is the most common cancer in men and the majority of people diagnosed with lung cancer die within 2 years.

Smoking is the single most important cause of cancer and is responsible for around 30% of all cancer deaths. In addition to the large number of lung cancers that are tobacco-related, a significant proportion of cancers of the mouth, bronchus, throat and bladder have been associated with smoking. Cigarettes carry a higher risk than other forms of tobacco.

Smoking was popular in the trenches in the First World War and British men continued to smoke heavily throughout the first three-quarters of the 20th century. During the last 50 years, high smoking rates have made lung cancer the leading cause of cancer death in men in Britain.

Bowel Cancer

Bowel cancer is the second most frequently found cancer in men and the chances of getting this type of cancer rise with age. Cancer specialists believe that diet plays a major role in the disease. Diets in westernised countries tend to be rich in animal meats, fats and alcohol, and low in fruit and vegetables, whereas the diets of people in less affluent areas of the world are more likely to be rich in fibre and low in animal products.

The prognosis for this type of cancer is very good if it is detected at an early stage when signs and symptoms first appear. The most common signs of the cancer, blood in the stools and altered bowel habits, usually have a simple cause, so immediate investigations are vital to rule out a malignant tumour.

Prostate Cancer

Age is the strongest factor in the susceptibility to prostate cancer. In other words, the older you get, the more likely you are to get the disease. Since we are now living longer, this in part reflects the increasing number of cases being identified. However, there is also a genuine rise in the number of people affected by the disease not explained simply by an ageing population. The likelihood of developing prostate cancer increases sharply over the age of 50, although a significant number of men in their mid-forties contract the disease every year.

As men age, their prostate gland grows. This is generally not a problem, but it can cause problems in some men because the enlarged prostate can press on the urethra and slow down the flow of urine, sometimes completely, causing discomfort and sometimes severe pain when there is complete retention of urine in the bladder.

Normally, cells of the body grow and divide under strict control. Old or surplus cells are programmed to die, and the number of cells in the body therefore remains relatively constant. Prostate cancer is a condition where the cells within the prostate gland begin to divide and grow in an uncontrolled manner. Why this should happen more commonly in later life is not clear but work is progressing which will enable us to understand more about this.

Pancreas Cancer

Unfortunately, this cancer remains quite common, especially in people over 60. Signs for pancreatic cancer are frequently non-specific to start with: poor appetite and weight loss are probably the first indicators, with pain in the upper abdomen and back. The later signs for this condition are very obvious – yellowing of the skin and eyeballs and darker urine whilst the faeces become pale.

Living with Cancer

Cancer can seriously affect your independence, whatever your age. Many people have lived their entire life in a very private and independent way. Watching this independence slipping away, if you have to rely on others to help you cope or make decisions, can be very upsetting and frightening. Don't be afraid to explain to those around you how difficult it is.

Often this loss of independence is a temporary situation, while you recover from the initial treatment for your cancer. When you feel better you can be assertive and firm in taking back control over your life.

During treatment, it is important to continue doing all the things that you enjoy. Some people find that keeping to as normal a routine as possible is very reassuring. Although energy levels may be lower during treatment, most people find they have 'good days' and 'less good days'. If you do the more energetic activities on your 'good days', you can have 'lazy days' on the 'less good days'.

If you have problems walking or moving around, it may be difficult for you to get to and from your doctor's surgery or the hospital. Sometimes your doctor will be able to call to see you at home instead. If you do not have your own transport and cannot travel by public transport to the hospital, ask your GP about other options, such as your entitlement to reimbursement of travel costs. Most areas have volunteer drivers who will take you to outpatients for the cost of the petrol, or your doctor may be able to organise an ambulance or ambulance car. If you need a course of treatment that involves attending the hospital each day for a few weeks, you may be able to stay in hospital instead of travelling back and forward each day.

As well as services, you may be offered equipment such as a commode or shower seat or minor adaptations such as fitting grab rails or a banister on both sides of the stairs to help climb stairs safely.

At various stages in the course of your illness you may be eligible for palliative care support from the local palliative care team as a free NHS service. Your GP or hospital consultant should be able to advise you.

Taking Medicines

You may need several different types of treatment to keep your cancer, and other health problems, under control. It may be difficult to remember to take all your medicines at exactly the right times, for example before or after meals. However, this is usually very important in making sure you get the full benefit from them. Your doctor may be able to have your medicines delivered in a daily dosing system box (such as a nomad or dosette box) which may make it easier to remember to take them. The pharmacist will provide a box containing all your pills, separated into compartments for the different times of the day and days of the week. You can see at a glance whether you have taken all your pills correctly.

Coming home from hospital can be daunting. If you are in hospital for any reason, such as surgery, radiotherapy or chemotherapy, make sure the nurses and doctors arrange all the support you need before they send you home.

The hospital will contact your GP to let them know that you are going home and the GP can then arrange for any care that you need. Services can include district nurses, Marie Curie nurses and Macmillan nurses.

District nurses can give nursing care such as dressing wounds. Marie Curie nurses give nursing care for a day, or overnight, to people who cannot look after themselves. Macmillan nurses can give advice on pain and symptom control and also provide emotional support to people with cancer and their families.

Ensuring that help and support are available at home is particularly important if you live alone. While you are in hospital, you will have people around to help you with even the simplest tasks. It is a big change to go from hospital to home and have to cope with housework, shopping, cooking and laundry, as well as looking after yourself and making sure you take all your medicines correctly.

Although you may be keen to return home as soon as possible, take time to think through whether you are fit enough to cope, and whether you need help with shopping or other tasks. It is usually much easier for the hospital staff to organise the help and support that you need, rather than risk a delay if your GP does it later. If you have family, find out what they will be able to do to help, as it is easy to overestimate how much time they have to spare. Once you get home, if you find you need more help temporarily, don't be frightened to ask for it.

Financial and benefits information

If you are living independently at home when your cancer is diagnosed, it is important that you have enough money to continue with your normal lifestyle while you are ill. Many older people worry that they will become a financial burden on their partner or children as they get older, and having cancer may make this seem more likely. This should not have to be the case if you seek out and claim all the benefits that you are entitled to.

If you are retired, you may be entitled to benefits in addition to your pension while you are ill. The Social Security Benefit Enquiry Line (see below) and the Citizens Advice Bureau (see Yellow Pages) can give you advice on benefits. If you are in hospital you can ask to speak to the social worker there, who will be able to advise you on benefits you can claim and help you to claim them.

Your local Age Concern may be able to give you advice on benefits and services available to you. They may also offer support, practical help, social activities and a range of publications and resources. You can find their details in the *Yellow Pages* or by calling the Age Concern Information Line (see below). The information line is a free telephone advice helpline which provides information for older people and their carers, friends and family on a wide range of subjects, from locating your local age concern, to advice on benefits and care arrangements. You can also order up to 5 free fact sheets on a range of subjects. All calls are confidential as are any personal details you may be asked to supply.

Macmillan Cancer Relief provides grants and financial help to people affected by cancer. A book called '*A guide to grants for individuals in need*' can help you to find other sources of financial support. The book is available from bookshops or libraries.

Each area of the UK has Patient Advocacy Liaison Services (PALS) which can put you in touch with local independent sources of advice on benefits and other aspects of your illness. Your doctor or nurse can tell you how to contact them.

Caring for someone with cancer

Although much of this book has been written for men who are trying to prevent cancer, or for those who have had a diagnosis of cancer, it is recognised that it might be also be useful for those who are caring for an older man with cancer.

As a carer for someone with cancer, you have an extremely important role in helping to maintain their quality of life as you support them through this difficult time. There is no one right way to deal with living with cancer. You can only do what is right for you. In the same way there are no magic phrases, or approaches, which are the correct thing to say, or do, in all circumstances when dealing with a partner, relative or close friend who has cancer. Indeed, in this situation, the important thing is not what you say – but rather how you listen.

Caring can be very hard work, both physically and emotionally. If you have been caring for your partner, relative or

friend for some time, you may already be completely drained. It can be easy to carry on, ignoring how exhausted you are, because you feel that only you can do what needs to be done. Asking for help can be difficult and may seem disloyal. Any support is valuable when you are feeling under pressure, especially the undemanding type that comes from family and friends. Asking for help is not a sign of weakness; it is more an awareness that problems can seldom be solved alone.

If you are at home looking after someone full-time, you may not have much chance to go out or spend time with friends. It may seem easier to stay in all the time, especially if the person you are caring for is very ill and needs a lot of attention. However, it is very important to maintain contact with friends and make the effort to get out regularly.

If you take good care of yourself it will help to keep your strength and spirits up. If you don't want to take a break, then you can at least give yourself little treats such as:

- *Finding time to sit down with a cup of tea.*
- *Ensuring you have peace to watch your favourite TV programme.*
- *Having an early night with a good book.*

Carers UK offer local practical and emotional support and can be contacted on their freephone number (see below).

Conclusion

Growing older is inevitable, but poor health in old age is not. The good news is that many cancers are preventable and many can be successfully treated if detected early. Adopting a healthy lifestyle is an important step to take if you want to increase your chances of keeping healthy and avoiding diseases like cancer. Being diagnosed with cancer in later life is not all doom and gloom, many people are cured and others manage to maintain a virtually normal life while living with their cancer.

This information has been prepared using information from the 'Cancer and older People' booklet, available free to patients and their relatives from CancerBACUP at the address below, the Prostate Cancer Charity and the Age Concern book 'Caring for Someone with Cancer'; details of these charities are included below.

Further information

If you would like to know more, look at the Contacts section, or contact:

The Prostate Cancer Charity
The Prostate Cancer Charity was established in 1986 with the primary purpose of improving the outlook for the many thousands of men and their families whose lives are affected by prostate cancer.
Du Cane Road
London
W12 ONN
Tel: 020 8222 7622 (general enquiries and donations)
Helpline: 0845 300 8383
Website: www.prostate-cancer.org.uk

CancerBACUP
BACUP provides a wide range of publications on all aspects of cancers. They also have a team of trained counsellors with whom an appointment can be made to discuss emotional difficulties surrounding the disease.
3 Bath Place
Rivington Street
London
EC2A 3JR
Tel: 020 7739 2280
Freephone: 0808 800 1234
Website: www.cancerbacup.org.uk

Age Concern
For up to 5 free fact sheets, or to find your local Age Concern, ring Age Concern.
Information Line:
0800 00 99 66 (freephone) 7 days a week from 7am–7pm
To order the Age Concern book '*Caring for Someone with Cancer*' by Toni Battison (ISBN 0-86242-382-1), call 0870 44 22 120. The book costs £6.99.

NHS Stop Smoking Helpline
0800 169 0 169

Quitline
0800 002 200

Websites inspired by hundreds of ex-smokers in the UK
www.ash.org.uk
www.sickofsmoking.com

Carers UK
Offer local practical and emotional support.
Tel: Freephone 0808 808 7777

Pass Your MOT!

Early detection: Some regular DIY checks

> **STOP!**
> *Only a real dope keeps driving when the dashboard lights up like the Blackpool illuminations. Ignoring the body's early warning signs is an equally bad idea and could mean an early trip to the garage for some vital spare parts.*

Attend your MOT

The MOT test keeps your car safely on the road and can pick up faults before they become dangerous. A regular check-up by your own GP is not such a bad idea for you either as it can pick up potential medical problems. Some GPs offer basic screening services and it is a good opportunity to talk about any concerns you might have as well as checking out your risks.

Check your documents

Only one lady driver? Check out your family history of cancer especially if one (or both) of your parents suffered from a particular cancer at an early age (ie, before 60 or so). It's important to check with your doctor what you can do to reduce your risk. Screening may be recommended and can catch potential problems early. Most cancers are treatable when caught early, but remember, many cancers are preventable in the first place (see Chapters 1 and 2).

Keep a regular eye on your bodywork

Get to know your skin so that you'll more quickly recognise anything amiss such as any new lumps or growths, a sore or bruise that does not heal, a mole that changes in shape, size or colour or bleeds in unusual circumstances (see Chapter 9).

Be aware of how your balls usually feel and check them every month or so for anything unusual such as a lump, thickening or swelling (see Chapter 7).

Persistent backfire? Check it out

Take action if you experience any of the following for more than a couple of weeks:

*   A persistent cough or hoarseness.
*   Shortness of breath.
*   Persistent indigestion or difficulty in swallowing.
*   Significant weight loss (for no apparent reason).
*   Loss of appetite.
*   A noticeable, persistent change in bowel or bladder habits, for no apparent reason (see Chapter 6).

Many symptoms that might indicate cancer are also just as likely to be caused by a less serious illness. But it's always better to be safe. So go to see your doctor if in any doubt.

H44856

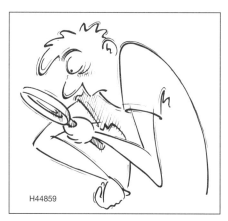

H44859

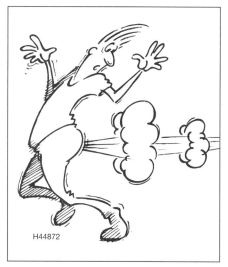

H44872

Coping with cancer

What to tell people

There are no rules about this. Taking your time and doing what feels right for you is the best thing. You know your own circumstances. Sometimes men do not include their partners or families in discussion with their doctors. They do this to save their family from unnecessary upset. However this may have the opposite effect. Loved ones are an important source of help – and they can be surprisingly strong on your behalf.

Feelings

Men respond in all kinds of ways to a diagnosis of cancer. There is no right and wrong way to feel, or for people close to you to react. Common feelings for everyone involved are shock, disbelief, fear and uncertainty, anger or resentment. These can lead to feelings of isolation and withdrawal. Some men feel 'out of control' when first diagnosed.

Asking questions is one way of getting back in control and you need to do this to make your choices work best for you. Your specialists will expect questions but it isn't always easy to know which are the useful ones to ask. It may help you take a list of questions like the ones below when you go and see your specialist or GP. You may find it helpful to have a partner or friend with you to help frame questions and remember the answers. Taking notes and asking permission to tape record consultations may also help you remember what was said.

- I would like my partner friend family member to be with me during this consultation. Is that OK?
- What are my choices?
- What do you recommend for me?
- Why?
- What stage is my disease?
- What do the results mean?
- What are the expected benefits of the treatments?

- What drawbacks or side effects should I be aware of?
- What happens in the future?
- How long will I take to recover?
- What is my prognosis?
- Will it affect my sex life?
- Will it affect my continence?
- What do I tell my sons/partner?

The information here is a good introduction but only covers the basic details. If you have prostate cancer you need more detailed information than you can find here – on side effects, new treatments or individual drugs, for example. Information is important when you have cancer and there are several organisations who can provide it and help with making choices. They produce ranges of literature, web sites and Helplines to make it easier for you and your family to discuss concerns and gather more information.

Abdominal pain

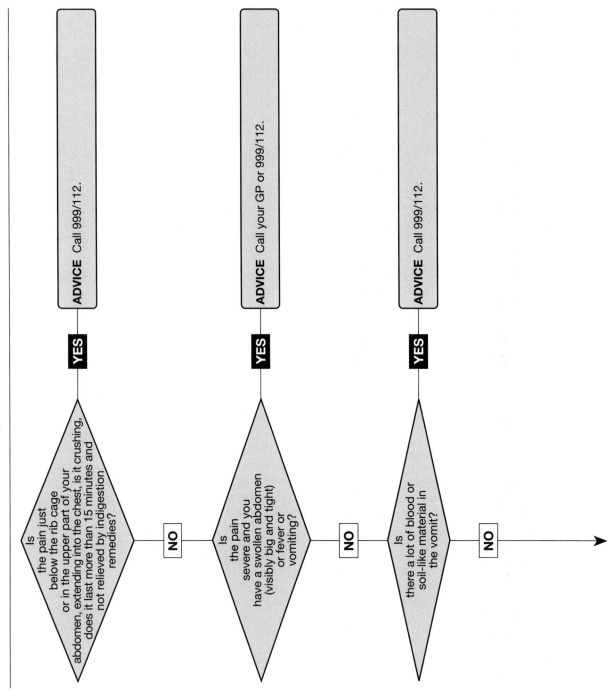

Is the pain just below the rib cage or in the upper part of your abdomen, extending into the chest, is it crushing, does it last more than 15 minutes and not relieved by indigestion remedies?

YES → **ADVICE** Call 999/112.

NO →

Is the pain severe and you have a swollen abdomen (visibly big and tight) or fever or vomiting?

YES → **ADVICE** Call your GP or 999/112.

NO →

Is there a lot of blood or soil-like material in the vomit?

YES → **ADVICE** Call 999/112.

NO →

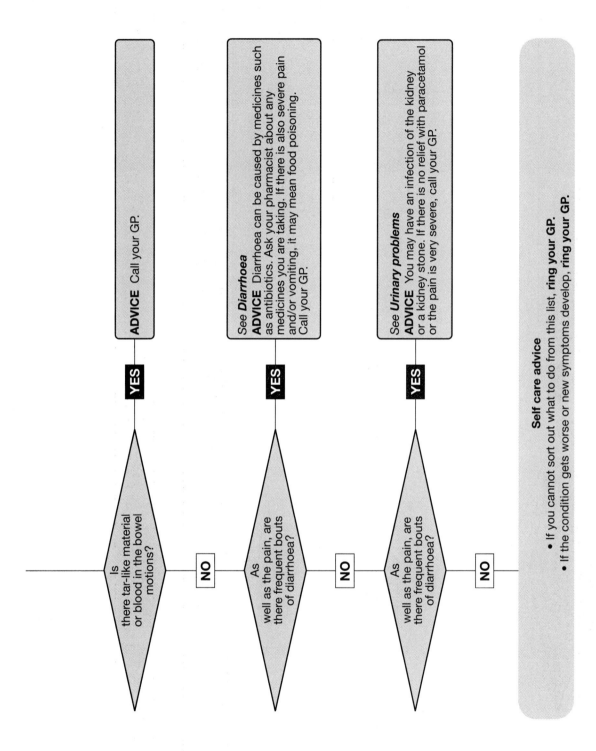

Is there tar-like material or blood in the bowel motions?

YES → **ADVICE** Call your GP.

NO

As well as the pain, are there frequent bouts of diarrhoea?

YES → See *Diarrhoea*
ADVICE Diarrhoea can be caused by medicines such as antibiotics. Ask your pharmacist about any medicines you are taking. If there is also severe pain and/or vomiting, it may mean food poisoning. Call your GP.

NO

As well as the pain, are there frequent bouts of diarrhoea?

YES → See *Urinary problems*
ADVICE You may have an infection of the kidney or a kidney stone. If there is no relief with paracetamol or the pain is very severe, call your GP.

NO

Self care advice
• If you cannot sort out what to do from this list, **ring your GP**.
• If the condition gets worse or new symptoms develop, **ring your GP**.

H44907

Back pain

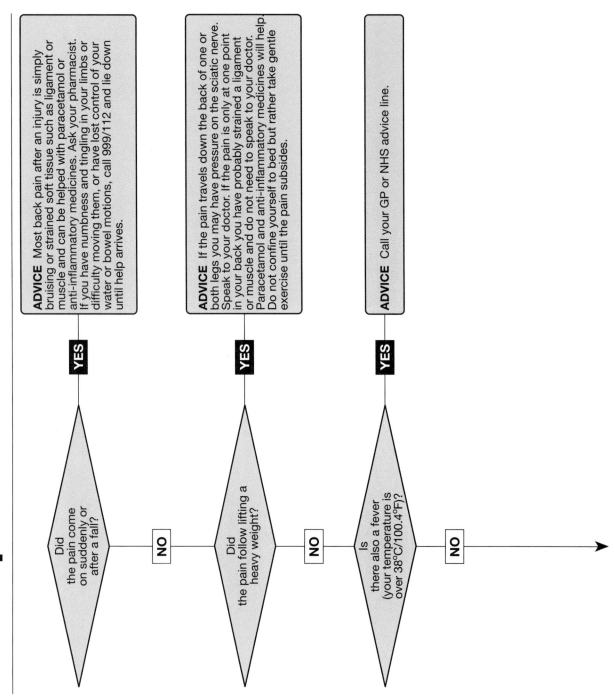

Did the pain come on suddenly or after a fall?

YES

ADVICE Most back pain after an injury is simply bruising or strained soft tissue such as ligament or muscle and can be helped with paracetamol or anti-inflammatory medicines. Ask your pharmacist. If you have numbness and tingling in your limbs or difficulty moving them, or have lost control of your water or bowel motions, call 999/112 and lie down until help arrives.

NO

Did the pain follow lifting a heavy weight?

YES

ADVICE If the pain travels down the back of one or both legs you may have pressure on the sciatic nerve. Speak to your doctor. If the pain is only at one point in your back you have probably strained a ligament or muscle and do not need to speak to your doctor. Paracetamol and anti-inflammatory medicines will help. Do not confine yourself to bed but rather take gentle exercise until the pain subsides.

NO

Is there also a fever (your temperature is over 38°C/100.4°F)?

YES

ADVICE Call your GP or NHS advice line.

NO

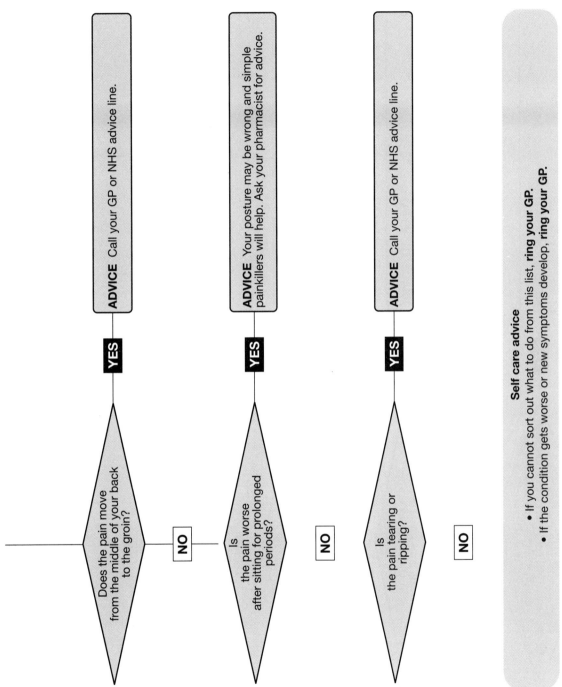

Does the pain move from the middle of your back to the groin?

YES → **ADVICE** Call your GP or NHS advice line.

NO

Is the pain worse after sitting for prolonged periods?

YES → **ADVICE** Your posture may be wrong and simple painkillers will help. Ask your pharmacist for advice.

NO

Is the pain tearing or ripping?

YES → **ADVICE** Call your GP or NHS advice line.

NO

Self care advice
- If you cannot sort out what to do from this list, **ring your GP.**
- If the condition gets worse or new symptoms develop, **ring your GP.**

H44909

Breathing difficulties

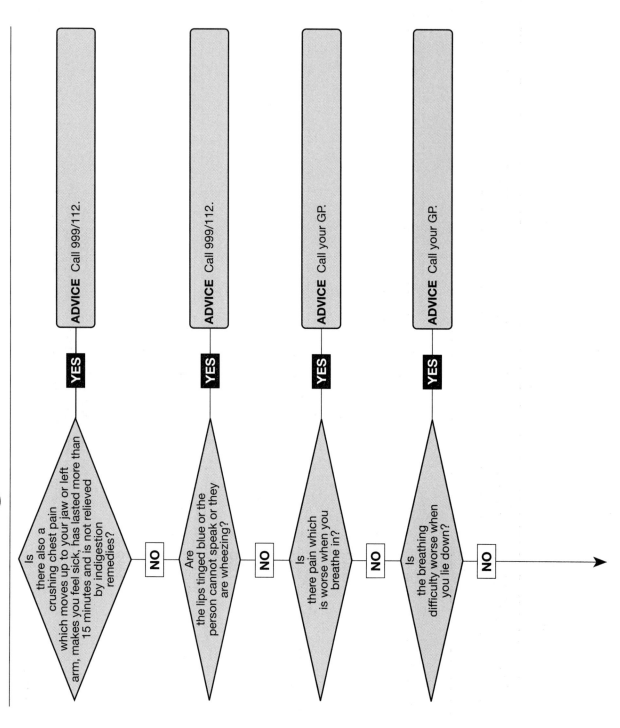

Is there also a crushing chest pain which moves up to your jaw or left arm, makes you feel sick, has lasted more than 15 minutes and is not relieved by indigestion remedies?

YES → **ADVICE** Call 999/112.

NO →

Are the lips tinged blue or the person cannot speak or they are wheezing?

YES → **ADVICE** Call 999/112.

NO →

Is there pain which is worse when you breathe in?

YES → **ADVICE** Call your GP.

NO →

Is the breathing difficulty worse when you lie down?

YES → **ADVICE** Call your GP.

NO →

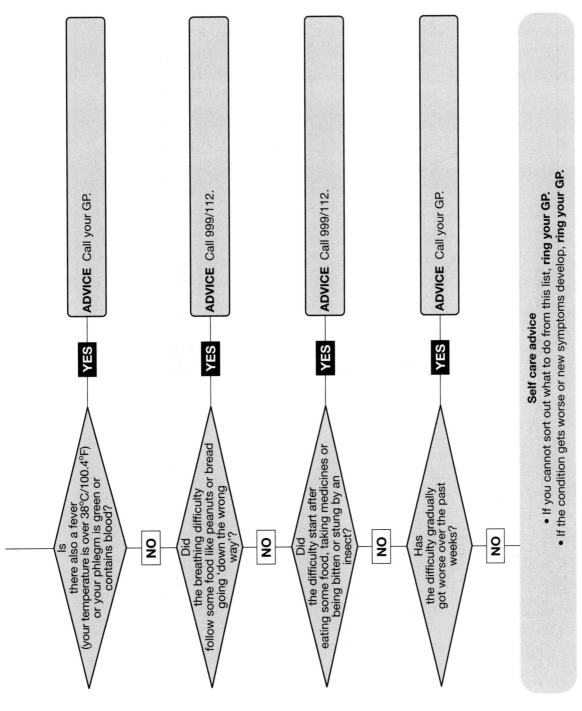

Is there also a fever (your temperature is over 38°C/100.4°F) or your phlegm is green or contains blood?

YES → **ADVICE** Call your GP.

NO

Did the breathing difficulty follow some food like peanuts or bread going 'down the wrong way'?

YES → **ADVICE** Call 999/112.

NO

Did the difficulty start after eating some food, taking medicines or being bitten or stung by an insect?

YES → **ADVICE** Call 999/112.

NO

Has the difficulty gradually got worse over the past weeks?

YES → **ADVICE** Call your GP.

NO

Self care advice
- If you cannot sort out what to do from this list, **ring your GP.**
- If the condition gets worse or new symptoms develop, **ring your GP.**

H44916

Coughing

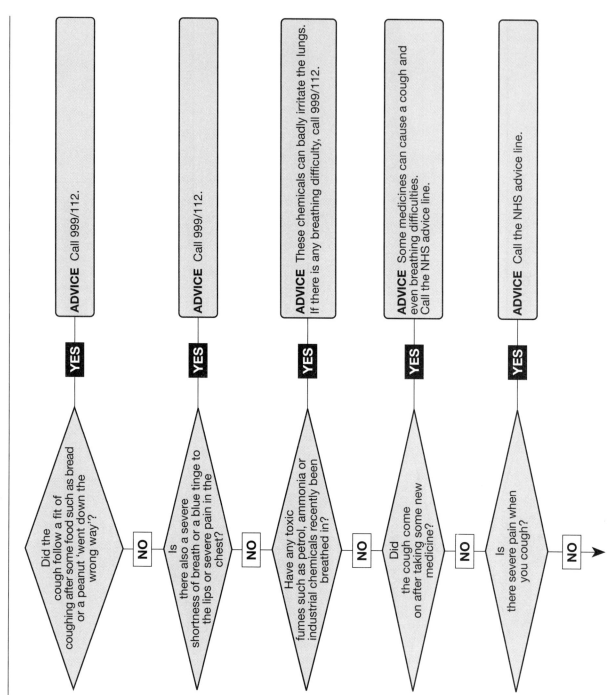

Did the cough follow a fit of coughing after some food such as bread or a peanut 'went down the wrong way'?

YES — **ADVICE** Call 999/112.

NO

Is there also a severe shortness of breath or a blue tinge to the lips or severe pain in the chest?

YES — **ADVICE** Call 999/112.

NO

Have any toxic fumes such as petrol, ammonia or industrial chemicals recently been breathed in?

YES — **ADVICE** These chemicals can badly irritate the lungs. If there is any breathing difficulty, call 999/112.

NO

Did the cough come on after taking some new medicine?

YES — **ADVICE** Some medicines can cause a cough and even breathing difficulties. Call the NHS advice line.

NO

Is there severe pain when you cough?

YES — **ADVICE** Call the NHS advice line.

NO

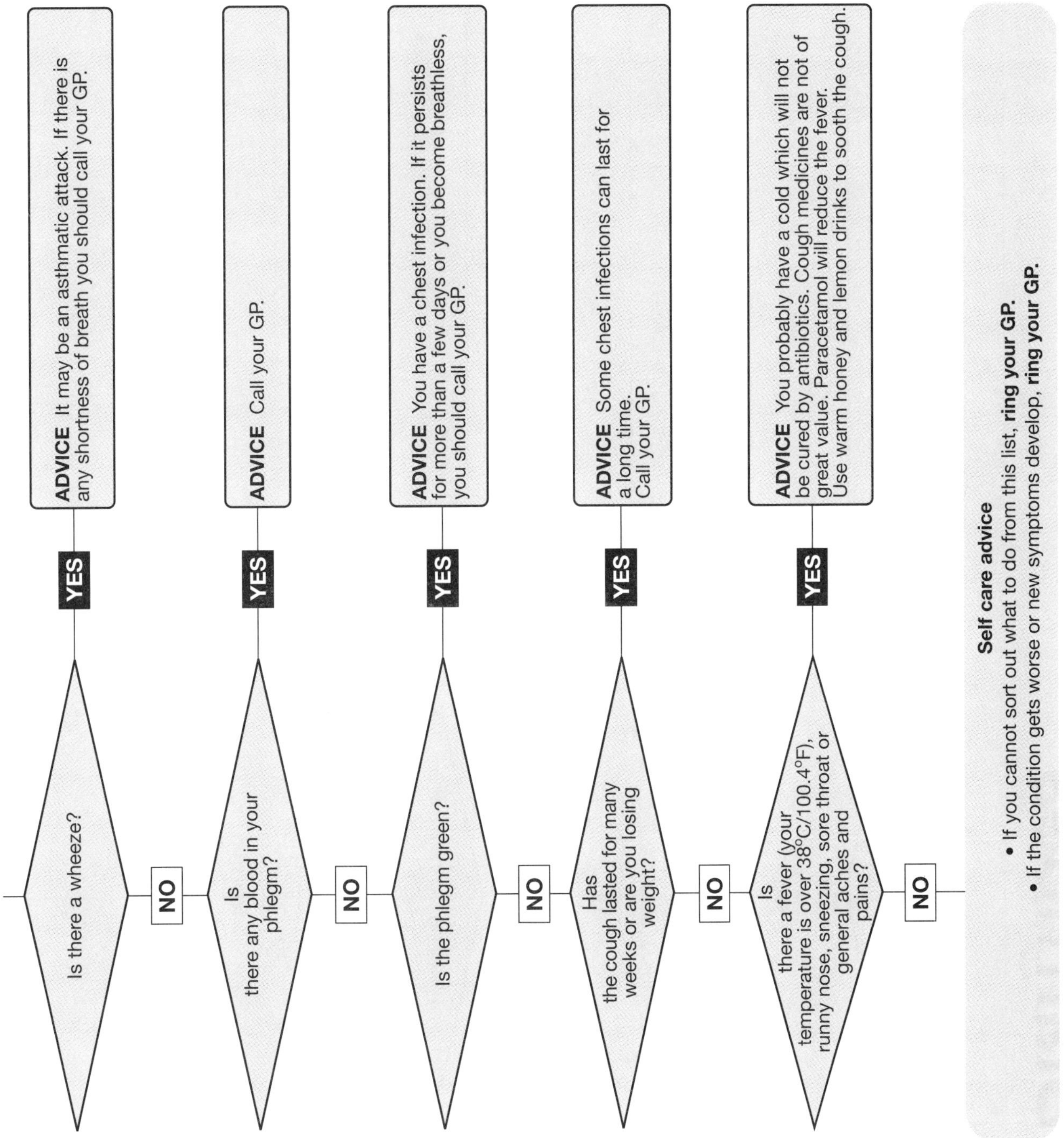

Is there a wheeze?

NO

YES — **ADVICE** It may be an asthmatic attack. If there is any shortness of breath you should call your GP.

Is there any blood in your phlegm?

NO

YES — **ADVICE** Call your GP.

Is the phlegm green?

NO

YES — **ADVICE** You have a chest infection. If it persists for more than a few days or you become breathless, you should call your GP.

Has the cough lasted for many weeks or are you losing weight?

NO

YES — **ADVICE** Some chest infections can last for a long time. Call your GP.

Is there a fever (your temperature is over 38°C/100.4°F), runny nose, sneezing, sore throat or general aches and pains?

NO

YES — **ADVICE** You probably have a cold which will not be cured by antibiotics. Cough medicines are not of great value. Paracetamol will reduce the fever. Use warm honey and lemon drinks to sooth the cough.

Self care advice

- If you cannot sort out what to do from this list, **ring your GP.**
- If the condition gets worse or new symptoms develop, **ring your GP.**

H44914

Diarrhoea

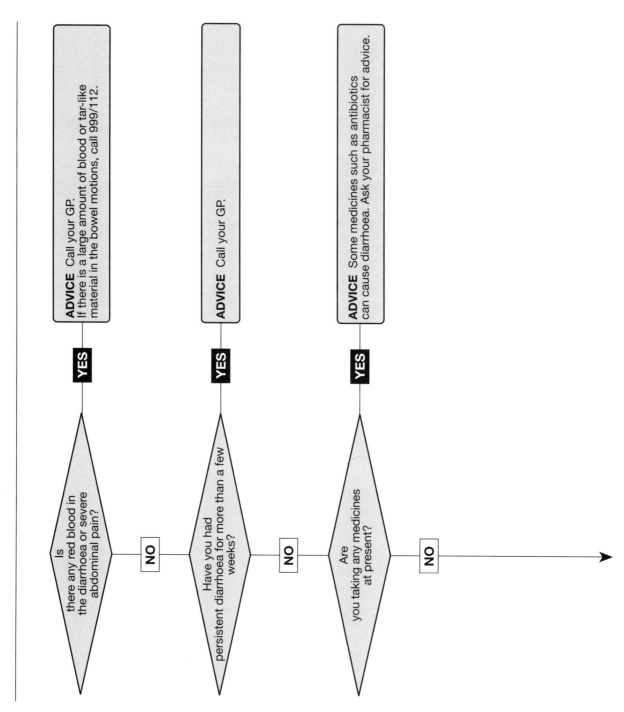

Is there any red blood in the diarrhoea or severe abdominal pain?

YES → **ADVICE** Call your GP. If there is a large amount of blood or tar-like material in the bowel motions, call 999/112.

NO

Have you had persistent diarrhoea for more than a few weeks?

YES → **ADVICE** Call your GP.

NO

Are you taking any medicines at present?

YES → **ADVICE** Some medicines such as antibiotics can cause diarrhoea. Ask your pharmacist for advice.

NO

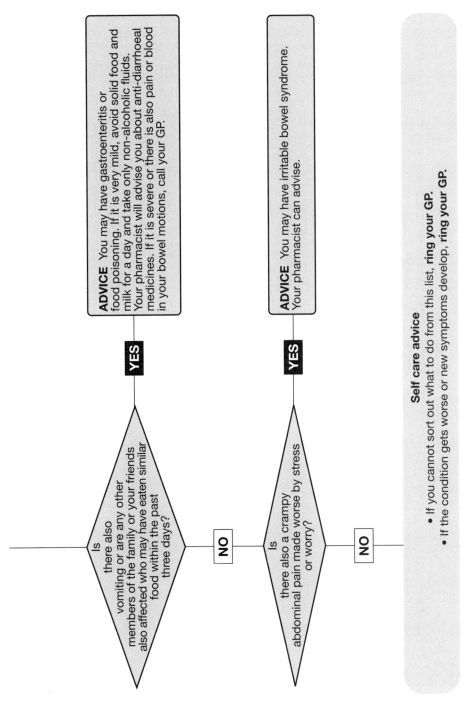

Is there also vomiting or are any other members of the family or your friends also affected who may have eaten similar food within the past three days?

YES

ADVICE You may have gastroenteritis or food poisoning. If it is very mild, avoid solid food and milk for a day and take only non-alcoholic fluids. Your pharmacist will advise you about anti-diarrhoeal medicines. If it is severe or there is also pain or blood in your bowel motions, call your GP.

NO

Is there also a crampy abdominal pain made worse by stress or worry?

YES

ADVICE You may have irritable bowel syndrome. Your pharmacist can advise.

NO

Self care advice

• If you cannot sort out what to do from this list, **ring your GP.**
• If the condition gets worse or new symptoms develop, **ring your GP.**

H44913

Eating difficulties

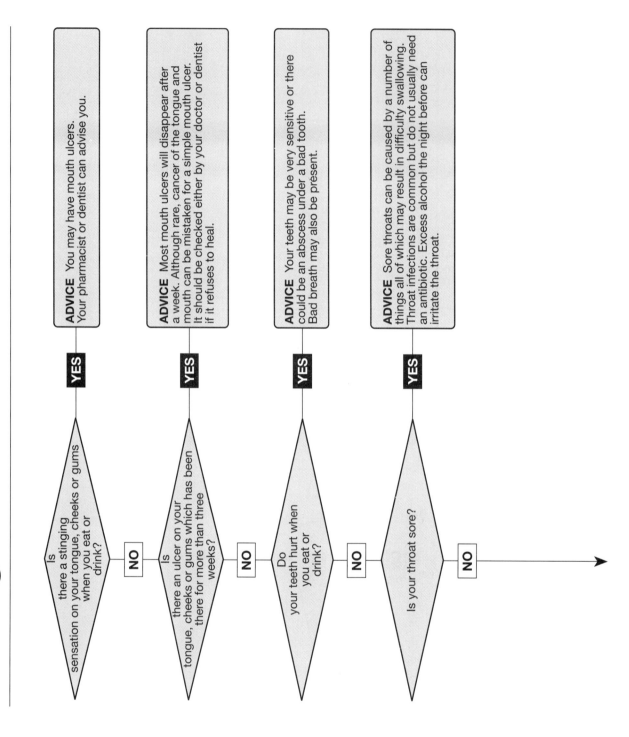

Is there a stinging sensation on your tongue, cheeks or gums when you eat or drink?

YES — ADVICE You may have mouth ulcers. Your pharmacist or dentist can advise you.

NO

Is there an ulcer on your tongue, cheeks or gums which has been there for more than three weeks?

YES — ADVICE Most mouth ulcers will disappear after a week. Although rare, cancer of the tongue and mouth can be mistaken for a simple mouth ulcer. It should be checked either by your doctor or dentist if it refuses to heal.

NO

Do your teeth hurt when you eat or drink?

YES — ADVICE Your teeth may be very sensitive or there could be an abscess under a bad tooth. Bad breath may also be present.

NO

Is your throat sore?

YES — ADVICE Sore throats can be caused by a number of things all of which may result in difficulty swallowing. Throat infections are common but do not usually need an antibiotic. Excess alcohol the night before can irritate the throat.

NO

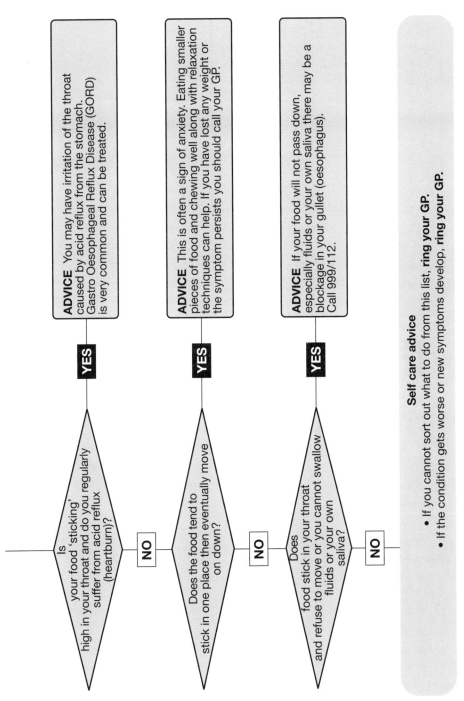

Is your food 'sticking' high in your throat and do you regularly suffer from acid reflux (heartburn)?

YES

ADVICE You may have irritation of the throat caused by acid reflux from the stomach. Gastro Oesophageal Reflux Disease (GORD) is very common and can be treated.

NO

Does the food tend to stick in one place then eventually move on down?

YES

ADVICE This is often a sign of anxiety. Eating smaller pieces of food and chewing well along with relaxation techniques can help. If you have lost any weight or the symptom persists you should call your GP.

NO

Does food stick in your throat and refuse to move or you cannot swallow fluids or your own saliva?

YES

ADVICE If your food will not pass down, especially fluids or your own saliva there may be a blockage in your gullet (oesophagus). Call 999/112.

NO

Self care advice

- If you cannot sort out what to do from this list, **ring your GP.**
- If the condition gets worse or new symptoms develop, **ring your GP.**

H44912

Headache

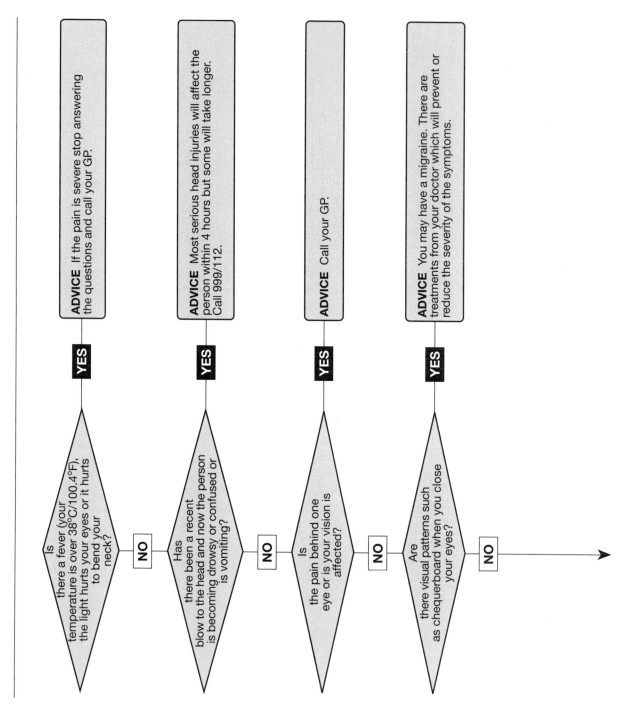

Is there a fever (your temperature is over 38°C/100.4°F), the light hurts your eyes or it hurts to bend your neck?

YES — **ADVICE** If the pain is severe stop answering the questions and call your GP.

NO

Has there been a recent blow to the head and now the person is becoming drowsy or confused or is vomiting?

YES — **ADVICE** Most serious head injuries will affect the person within 4 hours but some will take longer. Call 999/112.

NO

Is the pain behind one eye or is your vision is affected?

YES — **ADVICE** Call your GP.

NO

Are there visual patterns such as chequerboard when you close your eyes?

YES — **ADVICE** You may have a migraine. There are treatments from your doctor which will prevent or reduce the severity of the symptoms.

NO

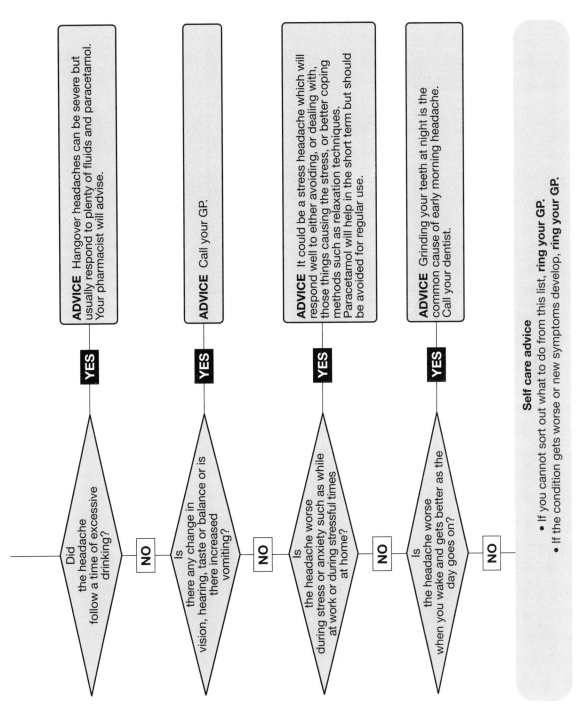

Did the headache follow a time of excessive drinking?

YES — **ADVICE** Hangover headaches can be severe but usually respond to plenty of fluids and paracetamol. Your pharmacist will advise.

NO

Is there any change in vision, hearing, taste or balance or is there increased vomiting?

YES — **ADVICE** Call your GP.

NO

Is the headache worse during stress or anxiety such as while at work or during stressful times at home?

YES — **ADVICE** It could be a stress headache which will respond well to either avoiding, or dealing with, those things causing the stress, or better coping methods such as relaxation techniques. Paracetamol will help in the short term but should be avoided for regular use.

NO

Is the headache worse when you wake and gets better as the day goes on?

YES — **ADVICE** Grinding your teeth at night is the common cause of early morning headache. Call your dentist.

NO

Self care advice

- If you cannot sort out what to do from this list, **ring your GP.**
- If the condition gets worse or new symptoms develop, **ring your GP.**

H44911

Hoarseness & loss of voice

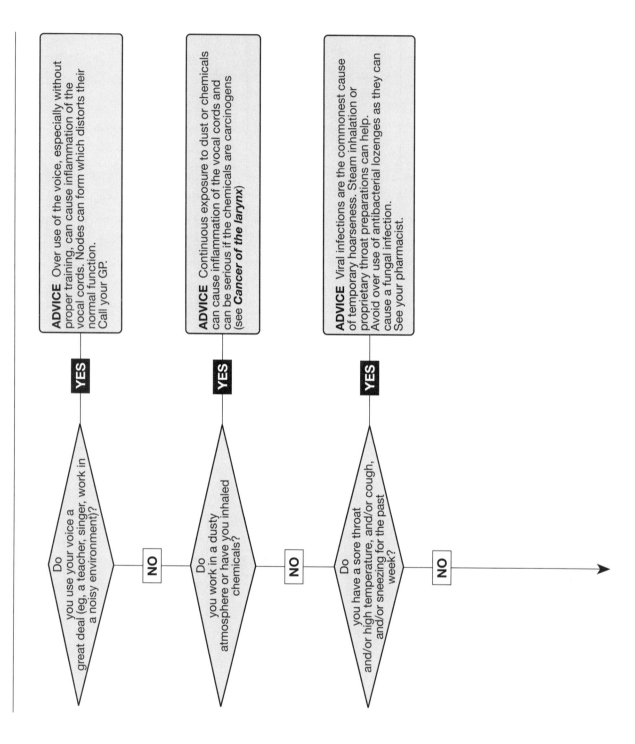

Do you use your voice a great deal (eg, a teacher, singer, work in a noisy environment)?

YES — **ADVICE** Over use of the voice, especially without proper training, can cause inflammation of the vocal cords. Nodes can form which distorts their normal function. Call your GP.

NO

Do you work in a dusty atmosphere or have you inhaled chemicals?

YES — **ADVICE** Continuous exposure to dust or chemicals can cause inflammation of the vocal cords and can be serious if the chemicals are carcinogens (see *Cancer of the larynx*)

NO

Do you have a sore throat and/or high temperature, and/or cough, and/or sneezing for the past week?

YES — **ADVICE** Viral infections are the commonest cause of temporary hoarseness. Steam inhalation or proprietary throat preparations can help. Avoid over use of antibacterial lozenges as they can cause a fungal infection. See your pharmacist.

NO

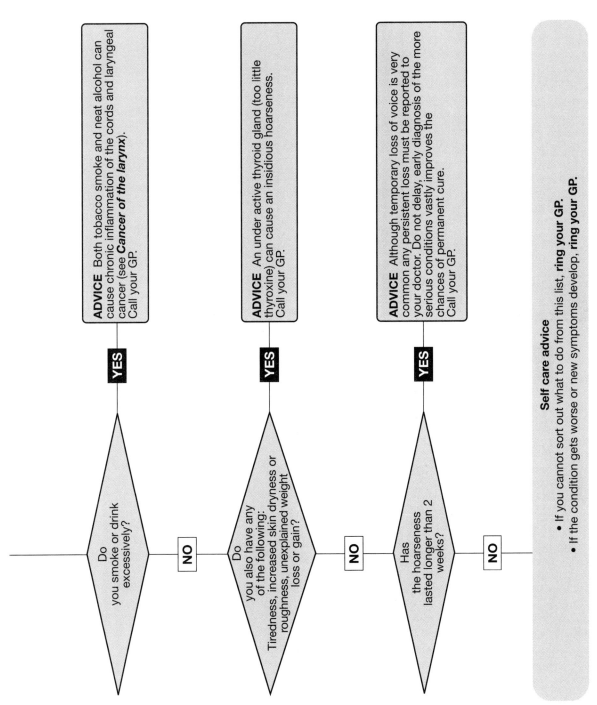

Do you smoke or drink excessively?

YES → **ADVICE** Both tobacco smoke and neat alcohol can cause chronic inflammation of the cords and laryngeal cancer (see *Cancer of the larynx*). Call your GP.

NO

Do you also have any of the following: Tiredness, increased skin dryness or roughness, unexplained weight loss or gain?

YES → **ADVICE** An under active thyroid gland (too little thyroxine) can cause an insidious hoarseness. Call your GP.

NO

Has the hoarseness lasted longer than 2 weeks?

YES → **ADVICE** Although temporary loss of voice is very common any persistent loss must be reported to your doctor. Do not delay, early diagnosis of the more serious conditions vastly improves the chances of permanent cure. Call your GP.

NO

Self care advice
- If you cannot sort out what to do from this list, **ring your GP.**
- If the condition gets worse or new symptoms develop, **ring your GP.**

H44906

Lumps and swellings

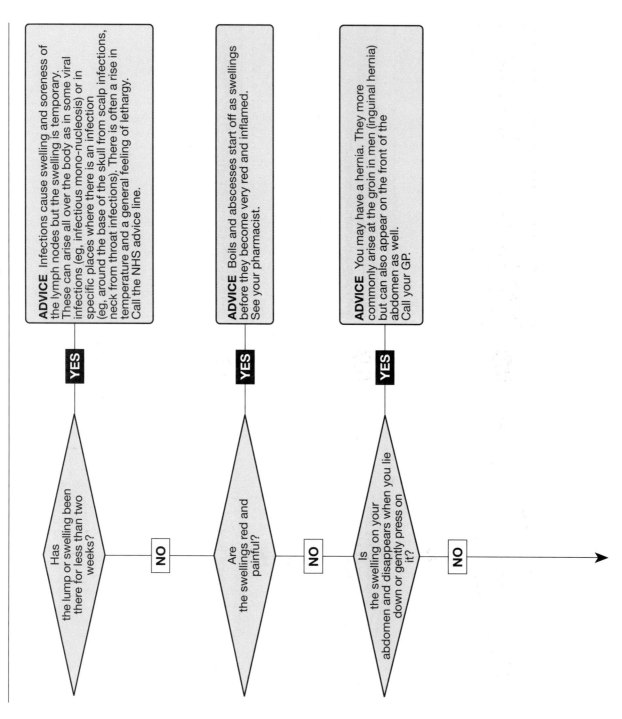

Has the lump or swelling been there for less than two weeks?

YES

ADVICE Infections cause swelling and soreness of the lymph nodes but the swelling is temporary. These can arise all over the body as in some viral infections (eg, infectious mono-nucleosis) or in specific places where there is an infection (eg, around the base of the skull from scalp infections, neck from throat infections). There is often a rise in temperature and a general feeling of lethargy. Call the NHS advice line.

NO

Are the swellings red and painful?

YES

ADVICE Boils and abscesses start off as swellings before they become very red and inflamed. See your pharmacist.

NO

Is the swelling on your abdomen and disappears when you lie down or gently press on it?

YES

ADVICE You may have a hernia. They more commonly arise at the groin in men (inguinal hernia) but can also appear on the front of the abdomen as well. Call your GP.

NO

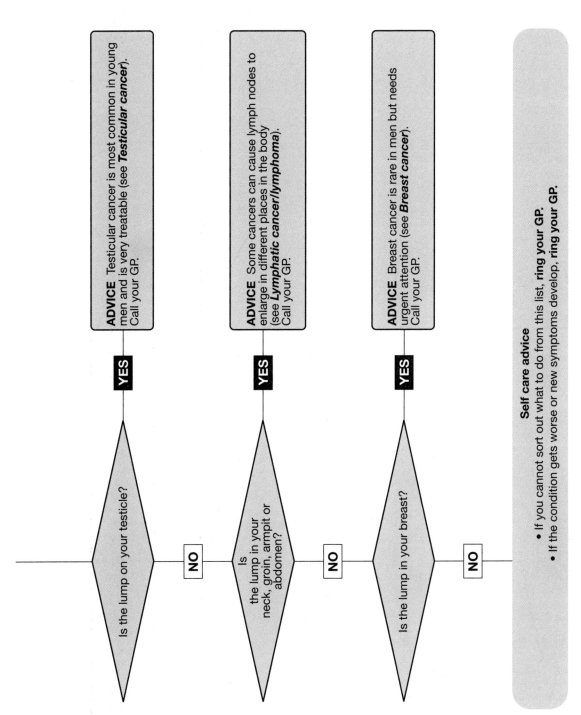

Is the lump on your testicle?

YES → **ADVICE** Testicular cancer is most common in young men and is very treatable (see *Testicular cancer*). Call your GP.

NO

Is the lump in your neck, groin, armpit or abdomen?

YES → **ADVICE** Some cancers can cause lymph nodes to enlarge in different places in the body (see *Lymphatic cancer/lymphoma*). Call your GP.

NO

Is the lump in your breast?

YES → **ADVICE** Breast cancer is rare in men but needs urgent attention (see *Breast cancer*). Call your GP.

NO

Self care advice
- If you cannot sort out what to do from this list, **ring your GP.**
- If the condition gets worse or new symptoms develop, **ring your GP.**

H44908

Testes

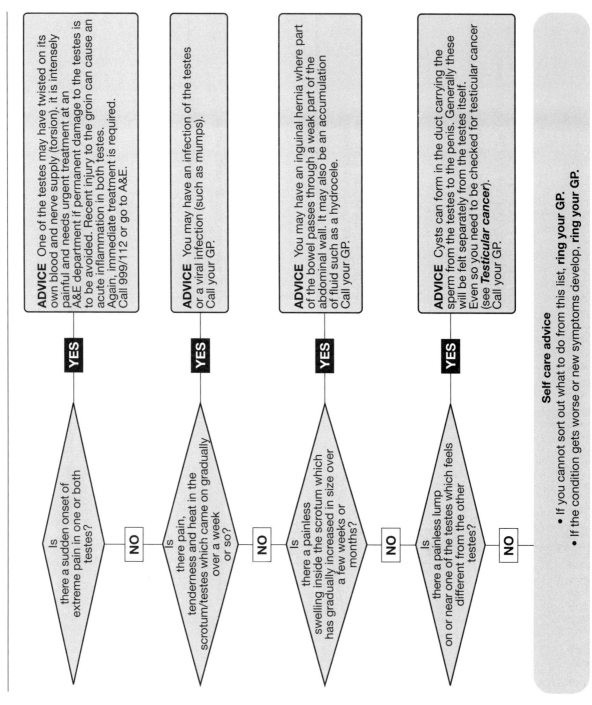

Is there a sudden onset of extreme pain in one or both testes?

YES → **ADVICE** One of the testes may have twisted on its own blood and nerve supply (torsion). It is intensely painful and needs urgent treatment at an A&E department if permanent damage to the testes is to be avoided. Recent injury to the groin can cause an acute inflammation in both testes.
Again, immediate treatment is required.
Call 999/112 or go to A&E.

NO

Is there pain, tenderness and heat in the scrotum/testes which came on gradually over a week or so?

YES → **ADVICE** You may have an infection of the testes or a viral infection (such as mumps).
Call your GP.

NO

Is there a painless swelling inside the scrotum which has gradually increased in size over a few weeks or months?

YES → **ADVICE** You may have an inguinal hernia where part of the bowel passes through a weak part of the abdominal wall. It may also be an accumulation of fluid such as a hydrocele.
Call your GP.

NO

Is there a painless lump on or near one of the testes which feels different from the other testes?

YES → **ADVICE** Cysts can form in the duct carrying the sperm from the testes to the penis. Generally these will be felt separately from the testes itself.
Even so you need to be checked for testicular cancer (see *Testicular cancer*).
Call your GP.

NO

Self care advice
- If you cannot sort out what to do from this list, **ring your GP.**
- If the condition gets worse or new symptoms develop, **ring your GP.**

H44918

Urinary frequency

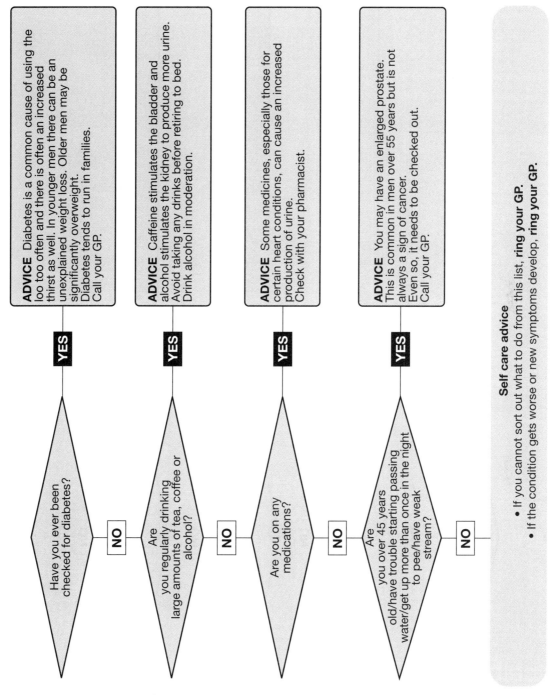

Have you ever been checked for diabetes?

YES — **ADVICE** Diabetes is a common cause of using the loo too often and there is often an increased thirst as well. In younger men there can be an unexplained weight loss. Older men may be significantly overweight. Diabetes tends to run in families. Call your GP.

NO

Are you regularly drinking large amounts of tea, coffee or alcohol?

YES — **ADVICE** Caffeine stimulates the bladder and alcohol stimulates the kidney to produce more urine. Avoid taking any drinks before retiring to bed. Drink alcohol in moderation.

NO

Are you on any medications?

YES — **ADVICE** Some medicines, especially those for certain heart conditions, can cause an increased production of urine. Check with your pharmacist.

NO

Are you over 45 years old/have trouble starting passing water/get up more than once in the night to pee/have weak stream?

YES — **ADVICE** You may have an enlarged prostate. This is common in men over 55 years but is not always a sign of cancer. Even so, it needs to be checked out. Call your GP.

NO

Self care advice
- If you cannot sort out what to do from this list, **ring your GP.**
- If the condition gets worse or new symptoms develop, **ring your GP.**

H44917

Urinary problems

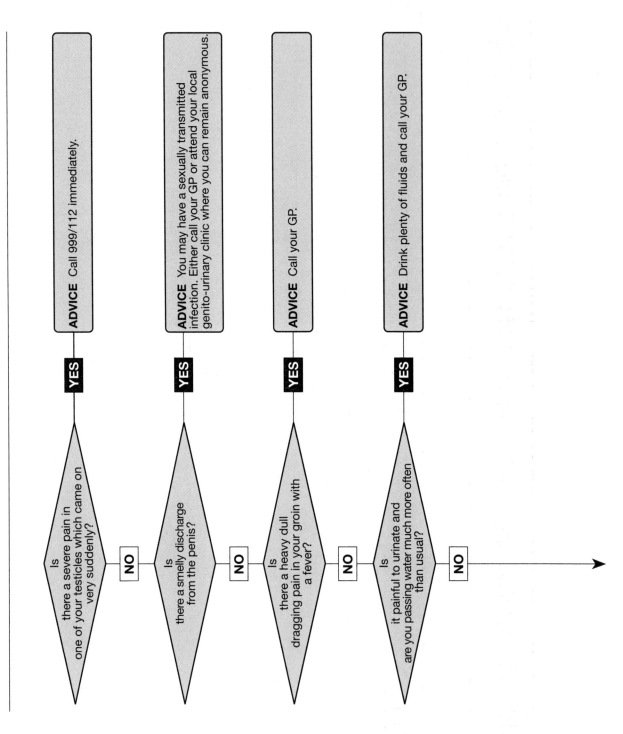

Is there a severe pain in one of your testicles which came on very suddenly?

YES → **ADVICE** Call 999/112 immediately.

NO

Is there a smelly discharge from the penis?

YES → **ADVICE** You may have a sexually transmitted infection. Either call your GP or attend your local genito-urinary clinic where you can remain anonymous.

NO

Is there a heavy dull dragging pain in your groin with a fever?

YES → **ADVICE** Call your GP.

NO

Is it painful to urinate and are you passing water much more often than usual?

YES → **ADVICE** Drink plenty of fluids and call your GP.

NO

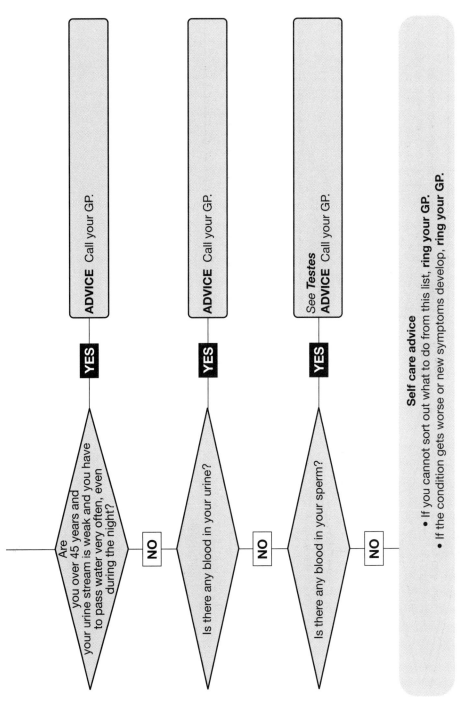

Are you over 45 years and your urine stream is weak and you have to pass water very often, even during the night?

YES → **ADVICE** Call your GP.

NO

Is there any blood in your urine?

YES → **ADVICE** Call your GP.

NO

Is there any blood in your sperm?

YES → See *Testes* **ADVICE** Call your GP.

NO

Self care advice
- If you cannot sort out what to do from this list, **ring your GP.**
- If the condition gets worse or new symptoms develop, **ring your GP.**

H44910

Weight loss (without dieting or trying to lose weight)

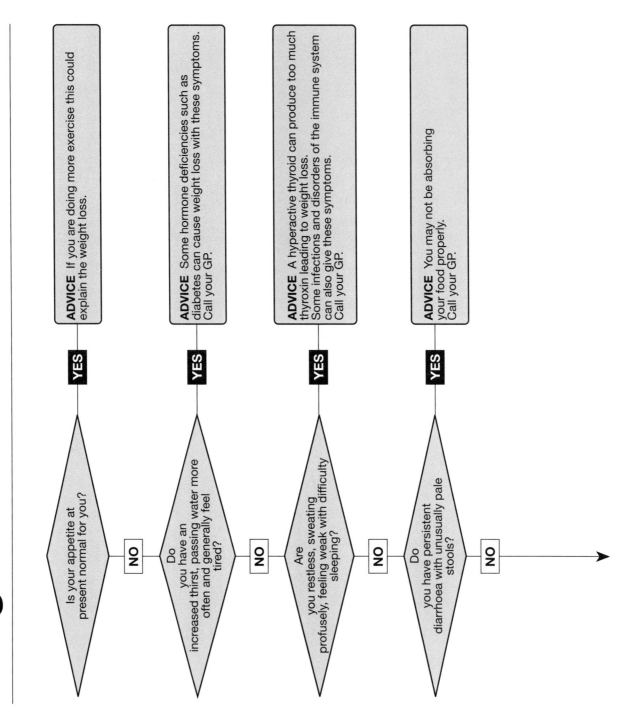

Is your appetite at present normal for you?

YES — **ADVICE** If you are doing more exercise this could explain the weight loss.

NO

Do you have an increased thirst, passing water more often and generally feel tired?

YES — **ADVICE** Some hormone deficiencies such as diabetes can cause weight loss with these symptoms. Call your GP.

NO

Are you restless, sweating profusely, feeling weak with difficulty sleeping?

YES — **ADVICE** A hyperactive thyroid can produce too much thyroxin leading to weight loss. Some infections and disorders of the immune system can also give these symptoms. Call your GP.

NO

Do you have persistent diarrhoea with unusually pale stools?

YES — **ADVICE** You may not be absorbing your food properly. Call your GP.

NO

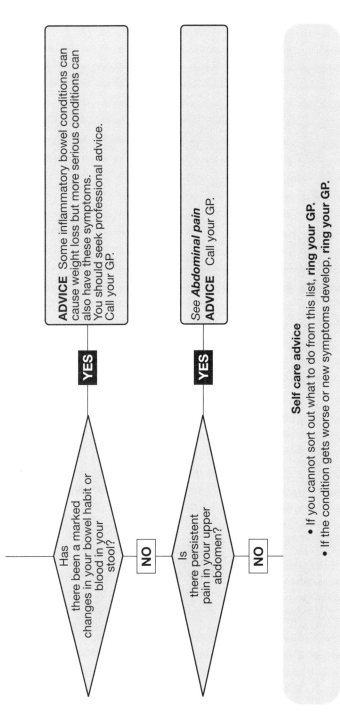

Has there been a marked changes in your bowel habit or blood in your stool?

YES

ADVICE Some inflammatory bowel conditions can cause weight loss but more serious conditions can also have these symptoms. You should seek professional advice. Call your GP.

NO

Is there persistent pain in your upper abdomen?

YES

See **Abdominal pain**
ADVICE Call your GP.

NO

Self care advice

- If you cannot sort out what to do from this list, **ring your GP.**
- If the condition gets worse or new symptoms develop, **ring your GP.**

H44905

Unexplained weight loss

(Over 4.5kg (10lbs) in 10 weeks without dieting or trying to lose weight.) Losing weight, or at least trying to lose weight, is very popular at the moment. This is perfectly reasonable if you are overweight, but there should be a good reason why you are seeing the pounds drop off. A significant loss of weight for no good reason is not normal. Increasing exercise will decrease your weight so long as you are not eating more than usual. Cutting down on alcohol if you have been drinking too much will also trim your waistline but if you are losing weight and cannot pin down exactly why, you should be aware of some medical conditions which include weight loss in their list of signs and symptoms.

Persistent diarrhoea with unusually pale stools may mean you are not absorbing your food properly. This may be due to an inflammation of the digestive system. Any marked changes in your bowel habit (how often you pass a motion) or any blood or tar-like substances in your stool, can be caused by inflammation or a tumour. This is not always accompanied by abdominal pain, although if pain is present, there is even more reason to get it checked sooner rather than later.

Contacts

Websites for cancer and men

There's a massive amount of material out there on the web but where do you start sorting through it? The information needs of a newly-diagnosed patient are different from those of someone who's had the disease for some time, the needs of a relative are different from those of a health professional.

So where do you begin to look for the information that you personally need? This section will help you to answer that question.

Search engine tips

The web is like an enormous library but although you're permitted to take out most of the books, there is no index system to help you find them. At best search engines trawl barely a third of the resources on the internet, often a lot less. So while your preferred search engine may be quick, its results are no better than those of an assistant with reasonable knowledge of a small corner of the library.

To get the best out of a search engine, try to be specific. Use the 'advanced search' option if available. This may allow you to select only UK sites or only those updated in, say, the last three months. This not necessarily because you are only interested in new information, but because you may well want to avoid dormant sites which are no longer being updated.

You aren't restricted to searching for individual words. You can use quotation marks to search for specific phrases. For example, to search for "testicular cancer". Also use + (plus) and - (dash/minus) to narrow down your results; note that the plus or minus signs must have no space after them. For example: 'testicles +cancer' will retrieve items that mention both testicles and cancer. The minus command might help if, for example, you wanted to find research by your doctor, the unfortunately named Dr Jekyll, but didn't want to be inundated with Robert Louis Stevenson references. You could try "Dr Jekyll" -"Mr Hyde"

A combination of the above can be very powerful indeed, enabling pinpoint searches. For example, "testicular cancer" +"Dr Jekyll" +"Belchester Bugle" could help you to track down that article your friend reckoned he'd seen in his local paper about your doctor and testicular cancer. This assumes, of course, that your search engine is aware of the Belchester Bugle website which, as we've already seen, is far from guaranteed.

Search engines do not all work the same way so a bit of trial and error is needed to work out how to get the best out of them. Some recognise certain short-cuts and not others. Search engines within a particular site – rather than a global search engine like Google – can be particularly frustrating as they have frequently not been built by search engine specialists.

Finding the right information at the right time is very difficult. I did an internet search when I was first diagnosed with Hodgkin's disease in the 1990s and was terrified by some of the results. Today, I might want to think about some of the issues raised but at the time it only made me feel worse.
Jim Pollard, editor of malehealth.co.uk and author of All Right, Mate? (Orion).

How to approach the internet

The internet is a resource that can help you get the most from a consultation with a health professional. It is not a substitute for a professional consultation. These websites are listed for information only and neither the author nor the publishers can accept any responsibility for their content.

That said, don't underestimate the value of the net. In a survey in the US in 2000, 70% of patients said that information they had found on the net had influenced their health decisions. Simply remember that if you choose to do so too, it is at your own risk.

Action Cancer
Provides full-time screening clinics for women concerned about breast and cervical cancer. Information, advice and evening clinics for men concerned about prostate and testicular cancers.
Helpline: 02890 244200
Tel: 02890 803344
Fax: 02890 803356
Email:
supportservices@actioncancer.org

Action On Smoking And Health (ASH)
ASH is a campaigning public health charity working for a comprehensive societal response to tobacco aimed at achieving a sharp reduction and eventual elimination of the health problems caused by tobacco.
Tel: 020 7739 5902
Fax: 020 7613 0531
Email: enquiries@ash.org.uk
Website: http://www.ash.org.uk

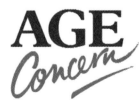

Age Concern
For up to 5 free fact sheets, or to find your local Age Concern.
Information Line: 0800 00 99 66 (7 days a week 7am–7pm)
Website: www.ageconcern.org.uk

American Cancer Society
The main US cancer organisation. Includes a facility for asking questions by email.
Website: www.cancer.org

Anthony Nolan Bone Marrow Trust
Searches for compatible bone marrow donors on behalf of at least 3,000 newly diagnosed patients each year. At any one time, we can be looking for donors for up to 7,000 people world-wide.
Tel: 020 7284 1234
Fax: 020 7284 8202
Email: healthgate@anthonynolan.com
Website: www.anthonynolan.org.uk

Asbestos Support Group And Mesothelioma Information Service
Helpline and other information and advice on mesothelioma (form of cancer usually caused by asbestos exposure, affecting cells lining the chest or abdominal cavities).
Tel: 0113 231 1010
Email: info@asbestos-action.org.uk
Website: www.asbestos-action.org.uk

Association for Cancer Online Resources
US-based, for people affected by cancer. Includes information and also mailing lists and discussion forums.
Website: www.acor.org

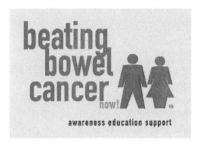

AstraZeneca
Website: www.astrazeneca.co.uk

Bandolier
UK site focusing on evidence-based health care. Requires a certain amount of prior knowledge to be used effectively.
Tel: 01865 226132
Email: bandolier@pru.ox.ac.uk
Website:
www.jr2.ox.ac.uk/bandolier/index.html

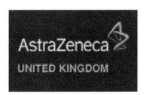

Beating Bowel Cancer
National bowel cancer charity.
Tel: 020 8892 5256
Fax: 020 8892 1008
Email: info@beatingbowelcancer.org
Website:
www.beatingbowelcancer.org

The Bob Champion Cancer Trust
Aims are to improve methods of detection and treatment, to identify cancer genes, and ultimately to eradicate male cancers.
Tel: 020 7924 3553
Fax: 020 7924 3042
Website: www.bobchampion.org.uk
Email: ask@bobchampion.org.uk

The Bobby Moore Fund
Cancer Research UK
Raises money for research into bowel cancer and aims to raise awareness of the symptoms so that people are diagnosed earlier.
Tel: 020 7269 3412
Email: bmf@cancer.org.uk

Brain Tumour Foundation
A national organisation for patients, their families and health professionals concerned with brain tumours. Provides information, booklets and a resource library. Is developing a support network of groups and individuals.
Tel: 020 8336 2020
Email: btf.uk@virgin.net

Bristol Cancer Help Centre
Pioneer of the holistic approach to cancer care.
Helpline: 0845 123 23 10
Tel: 0117 980 9500
Fax: 0117 923 9184
Email: info@bristolcancerhelp.org
Website: www.bristolcancerhelp.org

British Acoustic Neuroma Association
Support organisation for people with acoustic neuroma run by former patients and carers.
Tel: 01623 632143
Fax: 01623 635313
Website: www.emnet.co.uk/bana/

British Association For Counselling And Psychotherapy
Provides information on training as a counsellor, as well as information on counselling services available in your locality.
Website: www.counselling.co.uk

British Colostomy Association
Support, reassurance and practical information for people with a colostomy.
Helpline: 0800 328 4257
Tel: 0118 939 1537
Fax: 0118 956 9095
Email: sue@bcass.org.uk
Website: www.bcass.org.uk

Bristish Lung Foundation
The British Lung Foundation provides information on all forms of lung conditions. Runs support groups across the country.
Tel: 020 7688 5555
Fax: 020 8688 5556
Enquiries: enquiries@blf-uk.org
Website: www.britishlungfoundation.org

British Nutrition Foundation
Promotes health and well being by giving scientifically based information and advice on diet and nutrition. Cannot give individual dietary advice.
Tel: 020 7404 6504
Email: postbox@nutrition.org.uk
Website: www.nutrition.org.uk

CancerBACUP
Free cancer support service.
Tel: 020 7739 2280
Freephone: 0808 800 1234
Fax: 020 7696 9002
Website: www.cancerbacup.org.uk

Cancer Care Society
Provides free, confidential counselling, emotional support and practical help. Services include complementary therapies, befriending, an information library and a linkline for people with cancer to be put in touch with one another.
Tel: 01794 830300 (Mon-Fri 9am-5pm)

CancerHelp UK
Free service about cancer and cancer care run by Cancer Research UK. It aims to provide information on both prevention and treatment.
Email: cancer.info@cancer.org.uk
Website: www.cancerhelp.org.uk

CancerIndex
Links to cancer resources on the web by disease type and treatment. Looking up a particular type of cancer will yield a list of organisations and other resources on the web.
Website: www.cancerindex.org

Cancer Of The Eye Linkline (CELL)
24 hour helpline providing information and support for anyone who has lost an eye as a result of cancer or other trauma.
Tel: 01761 411055
Email: cell@zoom.co.uk
Website: http://www.cancerhelp.org.uk/pages.zoom.co.uk/cell/index.htm

Cancer Black Care
Aims to address the cultural and emotional needs of people affected by cancer, as well as their carers, families and friends.
Tel: 020 7249 1097
Fax: 020 7249 0606
Email: cbc@cancerblackcare.org
Website: http://www.cancerblackcare.org/

Cancerlink
Provides emotional support and information in response to enquiries on all aspects of cancer from people with cancer, their families, friends and professionals working with them.
Helpline: 0808 808 0000

Cancer Information And Support Services
Services for cancer patients, their carers, families and friends, and for health professionals. Helpline providing information on all forms of cancer, screening, treatment and prevention.
Tel: 01792 655025
Email: cancer_info_swansea@compuserve.com
Website: http://www.cancerhelp.org.uk/www.cancerinformation.org.uk

Cancer Specialist Library (CSL)
Covers the more common cancers in details. Most useful for health professionals.
Website: www.nelc.org.uk

Cancer Support UK
This Website has been developed to provide help, support and direction for anyone living with cancer.
Website: http://www.cancersupportuk.nhs.uk/

Carers UK
Offer local practical and emotional support.
Tel: 0808 808 7777

Fighting Britain's biggest child killer disease
CHILDREN with LEUKAEMIA

Children with Leukaemia
Tel: 020 7404 0808
Website: www.leukaemia.org

Christian Lewis Trust
Aims to improve the quality of life for children with cancer, and to provide emotional and practical support to affected families.
General enquiries:
Tel: 01792 480500 (Monday-Friday 9.30am-5pm)
Fax: 01792 480700
Family care services:
Tel: 01792 480500 (Monday-Friday 9.30am-5pm)
Fax: 01792 480700
Email: enquiries@childrens-cancer-care.org.uk

CLIC – Cancer And Leukaemia In Childhood
Helps young people under 21 years of age who have any form of cancer or leukaemia, and their families. Provides free 'home from home' accommodation adjacent to paediatric oncology units (ten homes at present).
Tel: 01173 112600

Colon Cancer Concern
Dedicated to reducing deaths from bowel cancer – also known as colorectal cancer – and improving the lives of those affected by the disease.
Tel: 08708 50 60 50
Website: www.coloncancer.org.uk

The Digestive Disorders Foundation
Information on a wide range of digestive disorders.
Tel: 020 7486 0341
Email: ddf@digestivedisorders.org.uk
Website: www.digestivedisorders.org.uk

Drinkline
Tel: 0800 917 8282

Electricity and Cancer in Men
Professor Denis L Henshaw
H H Wills Physics Laboratory
University of Bristol
Tel: 0117 9260 353
Fax: 0117 9251 723
Email: d.l.henshaw@bris.ac.uk

Everyman
Everyman was established by The Institute of Cancer Research to raise awareness and fund vital research for prostate and testicular cancer.
Website:
http://www.icr.ac.uk/everyman/

Expert Patient Programme
Tel: 0845 606 6040
Website: www.expertpatients.nhs.uk

Fatmanslim
Website: www.fatmanslim.com

Gayscan
Helpline for gay men living with cancer, their partners, families and friends.
Tel: 020 8368 9027
gayscan@blotholm.org.uk

Health & Safety Executive
Tel: 08701 545 500 (Mon-Fri, 8am-6pm)
Fax: 02920 859 260
Email:
hseinformationservices@natbrit.com
Website: www.hse.gov.uk

Help Adolescents With Cancer
A national charity offering counselling, group meetings and support for families and siblings.
Tel: 01616 886244
Website: www.mwmsites.com.\hawc

Ileostomy and Internal Pouch Support Group
Help for people with an ileostomy or an ileo-anal pouch.
Freephone: 0800 018 4724
Email: info@the-ia.org.uk
Website: www.the-ia.org.uk

Institute For Complementary Medicine
The Institute supplies information on qualified complementary practitioners, on complementary teaching institutions and on complementary medicine generally for use by the media.
Tel: 02072 375165
Website: www.cmedicine.col.uk

Institute of Cancer Research
Provides links to the widely-respected Royal Marsden Hospital and its patient information section, and to the ICR's own section providing an introduction to male cancers – Everyman.
Website:
www.icr.ac.uk/cancerinformation.html

International Myeloma Foundation
Dedicated to improving the quality of life of Myeloma patients while working towards prevention and a cure.
Tel: 0131 557 3332
Freephone: 0800 980 3332
Fax: 0131 556 9720
Email: TheIMF@myeloma.org.uk
Website: www.myeloma.org.uk

Leukaemia Care Society
Promotes the welfare of people with leukaemia and allied blood disorders; helps relieve the needs of their families.
Careline: 0800 169 6680
Tel: 01905 330003
Fax: 01905 330090
Email: admin@leukaemiacare.org
Website: www.leukaemiacare.org

Leukaemia Research Fund
Fighting leukaemia, Hodgkin's disease and other lymphomas, multiple myeloma, aplastic anaemia, myelodysplasia, the myeloproliferative disorders and related diseases.
Tel: 020 7405 0101
Email: info@lrf.org.uk
Website: www.lrf.org.uk

Lymphoedema Support Network
Advice and support for people suffering with lymphoedema (swelling of limbs or body due to blocked lymphatic drainage) following surgery or radiotherapy.
Tel: 020 7351 4480
Email:
adminlsn@lymphoedema.freeserve.co.uk
Website: www.lymphoedema.org

Lymphoma Association
Provides information and emotional support for lymphoma (Hodgkin's disease and non-Hodgkin's lymphoma) patients and their families.
Helpline: 0808 808 5555 (Mon-Fri, 10am-8pm)
Website: www.lymphoma.org.uk

Kidney Cancer Uk
Aims to provide UK kidney cancer patients and their carers with improved access to reliable information about kidney cancer and its treatment, and to establish a network of individuals and groups capable of offering mutual support.
Helpline: 024 7647 4993 (Every day 9.30am-9.00pm)
Website: http://www.kcuk.org/

Macmillan
Access to publications and information about support groups, and the opportunity to read other people's stories about cancer including patients, families, friends and health professionals.
Website:
www.macmillan.org.uk/cancerinformation

MARCS Line Resource Centre (Melanoma and Related Cancer of the Skin)
Advice line for anyone affected by melanoma or skin cancer and their families and friends. Information and advice about prevention and treatment.
Tel: 01722 415071
Website: www.wessexcancer.org
Email: marcsline@wessexcancer.org

Malehealth.co.uk
Promises fast, free independent information for the man in the street. The site is packed with information on cancer prevention.
Website: www.malehealth.co.uk

Marie Curie Cancer Care
Marie Curie Cancer Care, the cancer care charity, provides practical hands-on nursing care at home and specialist multi-disciplinary care through its 11 Marie Curie Centres.
Tel: 02075 997777
Website: www.mariecurie.org.uk

The Medical Advisory Service
This organisation provides a helpline staffed by nurses. They can give you information and advice on medical problems, including impotence.
General Enquiries: 0181 994 9874 (Mon-Fri 5pm-10pm)
Men's Helpline: 0181 995 4448 (Mon-Fri 6pm-10pm)

MedlinePLUS
General health site. The encyclopaedia section includes pictures and diagrams.
Website: medlineplus.gov

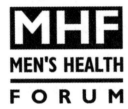

Men's Health Forum
Tel: 020 7388 4449
Website: www.menshealthforum.org.uk

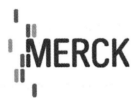

MERCK Oncology
Website: pb.merck.de

Move4Health
Move4Health campaigns and lobbies to make the physical, cultural, political and social environment more conducive for people being active. It also publicises how activity can promote health and wellbeing, contribute towards tackling the burden of psychological and physical disease to help reduce health inequalities in the UK.
Website:
http://www.move4health.org.uk/

The National Alliance Of Childhood Cancer Parents Organisations
NACCPO is made up of parent run organisations who have common aims of working together with families and health professionals to support children with cancer.
Website: http://www.naccpo.org/

National Association for Colitis and Crohn's Disease (NACC)
For people with Crohn's disease and Colitis.
Information Line: 0845 130 2233
NACC-in-Contact Support Line: 0845 130 3344
Email: nacc@nacc.org.uk
Website: www.nacc.org.uk

National Cancer Alliance
National membership organisation made up of users of cancer services (patients and lay carers), health professionals and other concerned individuals or groups affected by cancer.
Tel: 01865 793566
Fax: 01865 251050
Website: www.nationalcanceralliance.co.uk

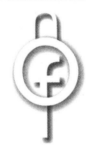

National Obesity Forum
Established to raise awareness of the growing impact of obesity and overweight on patients and the National Health Service. Membership is open to all healthcare professionals.
Tel/Fax: 0115 8462109
Website:
http://www.nationalobesityforum.org.uk/
Email:
national_obesity.forum@ntlworld.com

Neuroblastoma Society
Information and advice for patients and their families. Provides contact where possible with others who have experienced the illness in the family, for mutual support.
Tel: 01727 851818
Email: nsoc@ukonline.co.uk

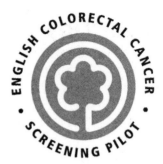

NHS Cancer Screening Programmes
Information on bowel and prostate cancer screening.
Website: www.cancerscreening.nhs.uk

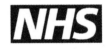

NHS Direct
Website that supports the NHS Direct telephone helpline service.
Tel: 0845 46 47
Website: www.nhsdirect.nhs.uk

No Smoking Day
Whether you are a smoker who wants to give up, looking to help others to give up on No Smoking Day, or just looking for more information about the Day itself you should find everything you need here.
Tel: 0870 770 7909
Fax: 0870 770 7910
Email: enquiries@nosmokingday.org.uk

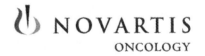

NOVARTIS
Website: www.novartis.com

Oesophageal Patients' Association
National support organisation for oesophageal cancer patients.
Contact Mr David Kirby Tel 0121 704 9860

OMNI
Free access to a searchable catalogue of internet sites covering health and medicine. Possibly most useful to well-informed search engine wizards.
Website: omni.ac.uk

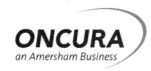

ONCURA
Website: www.oncura.com

Oral Cancer Prevention And Detection
The Website site has detailed information about oral cancer, causes, prevention, details of examinations, presenting features, and role of the health professional.
http://www.gla.ac.uk/Acad/Dental/OralCancer/

OralChemo.org
An online resource for patients and their caregivers, this sites provides information on all aspects of oral chemotherapy.
Website: www.oralchemo.org

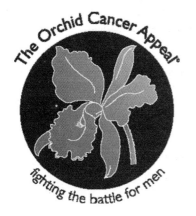

The Orchid Cancer Appeal
Tel: 020 7601 7808
Email: info@orchid-cancer.org.uk
Website: www.orchid-cancer.org.uk

Patients' Association
Represents the views and interests of patients to government, health professionals, managers and industry and campaigns for improved health services.
Patient line: 020 8423 8999
Admin line: 020 8423 9111
Fax: 020 8423 9119

People Living with Cancer
This is the patient information site of the American Society of Clinical Oncology.
Website:
www.peoplelivingwithcancer.org

The Pituitary Foundation
Information on pituitary tumours for people diagnosed with this type of brain tumour.
Tel: 0117 927 3355

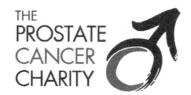

The Prostate Cancer Charity
Established with the primary purpose of improving the outlook for the many thousands of men and their families whose lives are affected by prostate cancer.
Tel: 020 8222 7622 (general enquiries and donations)
Fax: 020 8222 7639
Helpline: 0845 300 8383
Email: info@prostate-cancer.org.uk
Website: www.prostate-cancer.org.uk

Prostate Cancer Support Association
This organisation was set up by a group of men with prostate cancer in 1995.
Helpline: 0845 6010766
Website:
http://www.prostatecancersupport.co.uk

Prostate Help Association (PHA)
This organisation gives information on prostate cancer, prostatitis and non-cancerous enlargment of the prostate. They produce newsletters, books and run a support network.
Langworth
Lincoln
LN3 5DF

Prostate Research Campaign UK
Deals with all prostate problems, not just cancer.
Tel: 020 8582 0246
Email: info@prostate-research.org.uk
Website: www.prostate-research.org.uk

Quitline
Tel: 0800 002 200

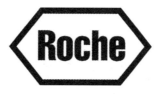

Roche
Website: www.roche.com

Rosemary Conley
Website: www.rosemary-conley.co.uk

Roy Castle Lung Cancer Patient Network
A network of lung cancer information and support groups throughout the UK.
Tel: 0800 358 7200 (Contact: Jennifer Dickson)
Fax: 01413 310590
Website: www.roycastle.org

Royal Orthopaedic Hospital Bone Tumour Service
(ROHBTS for Children and Adults)
Provides support for patients with bone tumours and soft tissue tumours.
Tel: 01584 856209 (Contact: Mrs Richardson)

Sargent Cancer Care For Children
Supports youngsters with cancer under the age of 21, and their families at home and in the hospital, from the day of diagnosis. Provides counselling and advice. Gives financial assistance to help with clothing, travel, fuel bills etc.
Tel: 02087 522800
Fax: 02087 522806
Email: care@sargent.org.uk

Save Our Sons – SOS
Testicular cancer information service, giving help and advice over the phone.
Tel: 01604 492610

Skinship (UK)
Helpline for people with any kind of skin problem including all types of skin cancer.
Tel: 01387 760567
Website: www.ukindex.info/skinship

Smoking helplines and websites
An advisor can put you in touch with your local NHS Stop Smoking Service.
Tel: 0800 169 0 169
Website: www.givingupsmoking.co.uk
Website: www.ash.org.uk
Website: www.sickofsmoking.com

Society Of Parents Of Children With Cancer (SPOCC)
A self-help group for parents providing social events and holidays for the children.
Tel: 01217 779468
(Contact: Ms Jo Taylor)

TAK Tent Cancer Support
Offers support and information for
cancer patients, their relatives, friends
and helpers.
Helpline: 01412 110122

Teenage Cancer Trust
Raising funds to build and equip 20
specialist units, to treat and care for
adolescents suffering from cancer,
leukaemia, Hodgkin's and related
diseases.
Tel: 0207 436 2877
Fax: 0207 637 4302
Email: tct@teencancer.bdx.co.uk

Tenovus Cancer Information Centre
Provides emotional support and
information on all aspects of cancer for
patients and their families.
Freephone Helpline: 0808 808 1010
(Mon-Fri 9am-4.30pm answerphone
service)
Website: www.tenovus.org.uk

UK Brain Tumour Society
Provides information, advice and
support for anyone directly or indirectly
affected by brain tumours.
Tel: 01293 781479
Fax: 01293 820720
Website: www.braintumour.org
Email: info@braintumour.org

Weight Watchers
Website: www.weightwatchers.com

WHCS Therapeutic Cancer Care
Advice, cancer care and complementary
therapies for people with a diagnosis of
cancer. Offer advice on cancer care,
health, terminal illness, bereavement and
other issues.
Tel: 0151 604 7316
Email: whcs.ttc@virgin.net
Website: www.wirralholistic.org.uk

WCT phoneline for men with cancer
(formerly Mind Over Matter)
Providing the opportunity to talk to
someone who has been through the
diagnosis and treatment of testicular
cancer.
Tel: 02386 775611
Fax: 02380 672266

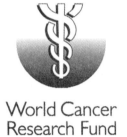

World Cancer
Research Fund

World Cancer Research Fund
Dedicated to the prevention of cancer
through healthy diets and associated
lifestyles.
Website: www.wcrf-uk.org

Banks, Ian *Ask Dr Ian about Men's Health* (The Blackstaff Press; Belfast, 1997)

Banks, Ian *The Man Manual* (Haynes Publishing; 2002)

Banks, Ian *The Trouble With Men* (BBC; 1997)

Banks, Ian *Get Fit With Brittas* (BBC; 1998)

Banks, Ian *The NHS Direct Healthcare Guide* (Radcliffe Press; 2000)

Baker, Peter *Real Health for Men* (Vega; 2002)

Beare, Helen and Priddy, Neil *The Cancer Guide for Men* (Sheldon Press; London, 1999)

Bradford, Nikki *Men's Health Matters: The Complete A-Z of Male Health* (Vermilion; London, 1995)

Brewer, Sarah *The Complete Book of Men's Health* (Thorsons; London, 1995)

Carroll, Steve *The Which? Guide to Men's Health* (Which?; London, 1999)

Cooper, Mick and Baker, Peter *The MANual: The Complete Man's Guide to Life* (Thorsons; London,1996)

Diagram Group, The *Man's Body: An Owner's Manual* (Wordsworth Editions; Ware, Hertfordshire, 1998)

Diamond, John *C Because Cowards get Cancer too* (Vermilion; London, 1999)

Egger, Garry *Trim For Life: 201 tips for effective weight control* (Allen & Unwin; St Leonards, Australia, 1997)

Finegan, Wesley C *Trust Me I'm a Cancer Patient* (Radcliffe Medical Press, 2004)

Inlander, Charles B. et al. *Men's Health and Wellness Encyclopaedia* (Macmillan; New York, 1998)

Korda, Michael *Man to Man: Surviving Prostate Cancer* (Warner Books; London, 1998).

Pollard, Jim *All right, Mate?* (Orion, 1999)

Martin, Paul *The Sickening Mind: Brain, Behaviour, Immunity and Disease* (Flamingo; London, 1997)

Ornish, Dean *Love and Survival: The Scientific Basis for the Healing Power of Intimacy* (HarperCollins; New York, 1998)

Cancer quacks

All it takes is a quick look at the internet, on an auction site or a search engine, or in the papers or glossy magazines to find thousands of references to alternative cancer cures. Beware! Many have outlandish names, and attractive presentations, with highly convincing statistics and quotations, but most will do no good, some will do harm, and more importantly they may procrastinate and delay the start of genuine, tried and tested medical and surgical treatments, possibly costing lives.

It is not surprising that unscrupulous people have a desire to make money from the misfortunes of others; there will always be cancer victims, and because of the nature of the condition, sufferers will always be desperate to find a cure, whatever the cost, and however bizarre the treatment; "it's a long shot, but it's worth it". An estimated $3-4 billion is spent on cancer quackery per year in the USA, compared to $1 billion budget for the National Cancer Institute. Up to 30% of American cancer patients attempt quack remedies, and three out of ten Americans believe that the government and doctors withhold effective therapies from the public.

The public is now well protected against fraudulent claims, but there are still individuals, methods and theories that slip through the net; theories such as 'intestinal flukes' being the cause of all cancers, and amazing Heath Robinson machines which guarantee a cure. There are said to be three distinct varieties of cancer quack: 'charlatans', 'huckster' and 'cranks'. Charlatans are fakes who make money by selling preposterous remedies to the unsuspecting public. Hucksters peddle bargain priced remedies, often from the back of a wagon, regardless of the suitability or effect; and cranks genuinely and sincerely believe in the remedies they sell, even though to the rest of us they may look completely ridiculous.

There may well be a grain of truth in some theories; who knows if a certain cactus or tree bark has properties which prevent cancer; but until something has been thoroughly researched it is best to avoid it.

There is nothing new about members of the public being misled by members of the medical profession, either genuine or bogus. There have been charlatans, hucksters and cranks around for thousands of years preying on gullible individuals, and making a quick buck.

Faith healers claim success in treating all manner of ills including cancer; one of the most celebrated was Valentine Greatrakes, the 'stroker' who, in the 1640s was inspired by a dream to cure almost every known malady using the gift of stroking. The Earl of Sandwich had healing powers; some people failed to respond to his 'curative touch', but that was, of course 'their own fault'. Later, in the 1890s Francis Schlatter cured hundreds of cancers each day, by standing behind a picket fence, touching the thousands of people who came each day who filed past on the other side of the fence. Those people who were unable to attend to be touched were still cured of their tumours when their very own 'blessed handkerchief' appeared in the mail.

A less comfortable form of faith healing was 'bone-setting', a forerunner of osteopathy, which worked on the theory that all illnesses, including cancers, were caused by dislocation of bones, which caused pressure on nerves and 'obstruction to the flow of life forces' through them. The noise during treatment was said to be like 'crushing an old basket'.

In the 1740s an old woman called Bridget Bostock cured 'the blind, the deaf, the lame of all sorts, the rheumatic, King's Evil, hysteric fits, falling fits, shortness of breath, dropsy, palsy, leprosy, cancers, and, in short, almost everything except the French disease, which she will not meddle with'. She accomplished her cures by praying over her patients and stroking them with her fasting spittle as the latter had to contain no trace of food. It was said that no one failed to recover.

In 1796, Dr Elisha Perkins from Connecticut patented his 'tractors'. The tractors consisted of a pair of metal rods about 4 inches in length, flat on one surface and rounded on the other. Rods were drawn over an affected area of swelling or inflammation in order to draw out any diseased process with their electric and magnetic effects. Tractoration for about 20 minutes a day was recommended and guaranteed to cure tumours and most other ailments including 'chronic rheumatism, gout, pleurisy, erysipelas and tetters, painful lumps and burns, and indeed most painful kinds of affections.'

Perkins' son, Benjamin, came to England following his father's death and set up practice in London in 1797 and in Bath, and the popularity of the tractors grew. In 1803 a Perkinean Institute was opened in London followed by similar provincial establishments for people who were unable to pay for the experience of tractoration. These flourished for a time until it was discovered that wooden tractors painted to resemble the original metal ones were equally effective when accompanied by similar pseudo-scientific jargon. It was gradually realised that there was no electrical or magnetic influence associated with the tractors and by 1810 the fashion died. Benjamin Perkins returned to America with his fortune – said to be about £10,000.

Other alternative therapies were taking over from the 'Tractors' at that time. In 1812, the Medical Guide, for the use of Clergy, Heads of Families, and Practitioners in Medicine and Surgery, by Richard Reece, M.D. recommended:

For the treatment of cancer, "to rouse the action of the absorbents of the parts and to promote healthy mutation, friction is necessary. The morbid irritation should be allayed by extracting blood by means of leeches; by a sedative application;

and by reducing the general ignition of the system, if it should run high. The best local application is a plaster composed of mercury and a vegetable anodyne, spread on soft leather. Take of strong mercurial ointment, gum ammoniac, and extract of hemlock, of equal parts. The gum ammoniac to be reduced to a fine pulp by means of a little water, and afterwards the whole to be blended in a marble mortar. Over this plaster a dried hare-skin should be worn."

Perhaps the greatest period for quack remedies started in the late Victorian era toward the end of the 19th century. Newspapers were widely available allowing remedies to be advertised to a wide audience; scientific discoveries were occurring, so the public was open minded to new theories, and modern regulations hadn't been introduced to curb the sale of dubious items. Entire establishments were founded upon dubious claims for cancer treatment. The Park View Sanatorium was one such institution, where the remedy 'Cancerol' was used to cure a long list of cancers. The Berkshire Hills Sanatorium was founded 'for the scientific treatment of cancer without the use of the knife: The Largest and Best Equipped Private Institution in the World. For the exclusive treatment of cancer and all other forms of malignant and benign new growths, except cancer and tumours within the abdominal cavity'. It wasn't just the remedies, however, which fell into disrepute; the equipment itself was sometimes not what it seemed. The impressively named "Advanced Medical Science Institute" in Omaha was equipped with "$12,000 worth of wonderful electrical apparatus including an 'electro-oxygen' machine, with which in conjunction with the famous 'Friedman Serum' could cure tuberculosis, Bright's disease, Diabetes and cancer". Each piece of equipment was entirely worthless. Apparently knowing that they were about to be arrested, the proprietors, Dr E.D. Brantley and Dr X.W. Witman took 'a large sum of money from their patients' and fled.

The New York Medical Institute went one better. The State Department of Labor of New York described this particular swindle: " The applicant is ushered into a private office. He is placed before a large machine of complex appearance that conveys the impression to the ignorant patient of being costly and almost miraculous, and is examined by the physicians, who dramatically and with apparent emotion inform the patient that he is suffering from some dreadful disease, which, if longer neglected will result in death. The patient becomes alarmed and agrees to pay any price for a cure, which is guaranteed. It is unnecessary to state that the so-called examination and later 'treatment' are absolutely without merit. Many victims, having been robbed of all their money were found by reputable physicians to be suffering from no disease at all."

More and more Institutes sprung up, competing with each other for the most outlandish claims. A multitude of patent medicines and drugs were marketed at massive profit, with no benefit to patients.

- **Aqua Nova Vita***: a remedy for blood and gland disorders, hardening of the arteries, Cancer internal and external.*

- *Dr E.E. Burnside's* **PURIFICO** *for Cancer Tumor and all blood disorders.*
- **Hoods SASPARILLA** *for Scrofula, eczema, cancerous humours, catarrh, varicose veins and 'female weakness'.*

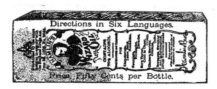

- **Hamlin's WIZARD OIL** *to check the growth and permanently cure cancer and prevent rabies.*
- **Lindsey's Improved BLOOD SEARCHER** *for diseases of women, malaria, cancer, sore eyes and piles.*

A tree bark called Cundurango was wrongly thought to have cancer curing properties; the deception was revealed in a poem published in 1877:

The morning sun was shining bright,
As lone upon old Georgetown's height,
A Bliss-ful doctor, clad in brown,
Desiring wealth and great renown,
Displayed aloft to wondering eyes
A shrub which bore this strange device,
Cundurango!

A maiden fair, with pallid cheek
With ardent haste his aid did seek
To stay the progress and the pain
Of carcinoma of the brain;
While still aloft the shrub he bore,
The answer came, with windy roar,
To Cundurango!

A matron old, with long unrest
From carcinoma of the breast,
This Bliss-ful doctor rushed to see,
And begged his aid on bended knee.
The magic shrub waved still on high,
And rushed through air the well-known cry,
Try Cundurango!

The evening sun went down in red-
The maid and matron both were dead;
And yet, through all the realms around,
This worthless shrub, of mighty sound,
Will serve to fill the purse forlorn,
And the cancer succumb "in a horn"
To Cundurango.

Even ointments apparently had the power to cure cancer:

- **Russia Salve** *for cancers, mosquito bites, swelled nose and ingrowing toe-nails.*

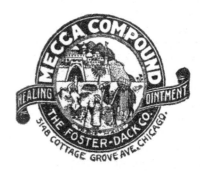

- **Mecca Compound** *for erysipelas, gangrene, blood poisoning, cancers, bronchitis, diphtheria, pleurisy, pneumonia, scarlet fever, smallpox, lockjaw, goitre, measles, tuberculosis and the early stages of appendicitis.*

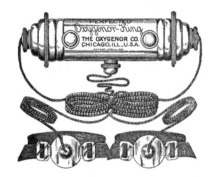

And a vast array of devices, ranging from the simple *Electro-chemical Ring;* an iron ring, worn on the finger, to Electro-magnetic belts and *Oxygenators,* and the infamous *Wm Radam's Microbe Killer.*

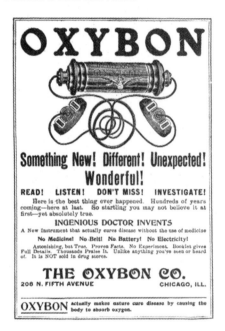

It's hardly surprising that these "cures" made a fortune for their inventors!

The authorities started to clamp down on fraudsters, helped by the American and British Medical Associations, who painstakingly analysed, and ridiculed the different concoctions put up for sale as cancer cures.

- **Mrs Joe Person's Remedy** *which modestly promised to cure cancer in its early stages, was 'a slightly sweetened water-alcohol solution of vegetable drugs, podophyllin and sarsaparilla'.*
- **Porter's Antiseptic Healing oil** *which 'removed tumors and*

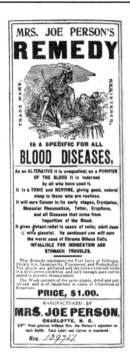

cancerous growths' turned out to be camphor and carbolic acid in cotton-seed oil.

- **Radway's SASPARILLIAN** *a cure for cancer, falling of the womb, paralysis and diabetes was an impressive 16.5% alcohol with arsenic and 'certain plant substance'.*
- *Similarly* **Raney's Blood Remedy** *was merely potash in syrup with 16% alcohol, but somehow managed to cure cancer, pellagra, female complaints, rheumatism, diseases of the kidneys, all blood and nerve diseases, and in addition was a 'nerve rebuilder'.*
- **Dr Sherman** *was fined $10 when it was discovered that his* **Compound Prickly Ash Bitters** *for gallstones, incontinence, dropsy and malignant diseases of the kidney, were 20% alcohol, and the daily dose was equivalent to an entire bottle of wine.*
- **Dr Shoop's Night Cure** *was a variation on a theme, being a suppository, composed mainly of cacao butter, which cured ovarian and other tumours.*
- **Dr Upham,** *despite his name, didn't sell suppositories, but a* **Valuable Electuary;** *an infallible cure for paralysis, apoplexy, piles, measles and tumours of the stomach. He was fined $100 for passing off cream of tartar as a universal cure.*

Some fraudsters, however, stooped even lower, and their methods were highly sinister and dangerous. *Tanlac* was a "tonic and system purifier" made by the Cooper Medicine Company, which genuinely had a tonic effect in many patients because of the main ingredient; 17% alcohol. Its publicity claimed "Tanlac is called the magic medicine... preserves your health, gives you renewed energy, brightens your spirits, lengthens your life." The theory was simple; every ailment including cancer, was caused by one thing and one thing only; Catarrh. Therefore an infallible treatment for catarrh, such as Tanlac, would cure all ailments including cancer. Many medicines and nostrums would prove their efficacy by including testimonials from individuals who had tried the remedy; these were usually fairly dubious, as they were paid for by the company, or exaggerated beyond recognition, or more often than not, completely fictitious.

South Hadley Man Relieved of Stomach Trouble Since Taking Tanlac the National Tonic 'I have gained 10 pounds' says Fred Wicks 'and my wife and son are also taking Tanlac and have been greatly benefited'.

At least the patient Fred Wicks did actually exist, as proved by his obituary, published in the same edition of the Holyoke Daily Transcript as his testimonial, May 11th 1917. He died of carcinoma of the stomach, two days before his testimonial was published, having taken Tanlac, a mixture of alcohol, liquorice and berries, instead of seeking traditional medical help which could have cured him. Far from being an unfortunate coincidence, Cooper Medicine Company became renowned for its so-called 'Testimonials from the grave' as more and more people died from the condition of which they had supposedly been cured, and were unable to contradict their glowing reference to Tanlac. L.T. Cooper was arrested in October 1914 in Lexington Kentucky.

Worse still was the notorious case of Dr S.R. Chamlee, the Cancer-Cure quack who defrauded the public for more than a quarter of a century. Known as a 'vicious, sinister parasite' he was

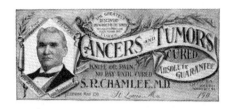

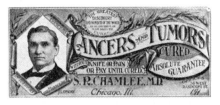

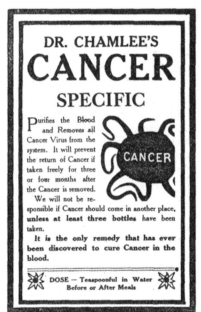

possibly but not probably. Of all tainted gold none is quite so dirty as that filched from the hopeless sufferers from civilization's most dreaded scourge" The least of his deceptions was his 'Cancer Specific' which he claimed killed 'cancer germs', but only if one drank at least three bottles. The very worst of Chamlee's deceptions was actually to perform operations on healthy people, whom he had convinced had cancer. He was known to operate on them with 'some such instrument as a pair of shears', and pack wounds with 'cloth smeared with some dirty greenish ointment'. He used no antiseptic techniques, and when these previously healthy patients were on the point of death from blood poisoning, 'to avoid unpleasant consequences Chamlee took the precaution to pack them up and send them out of town to avoid an inquest'.

But most impressively outrageous of all the claims for any cancer remedy

must surely be those made for *James A. Davis' HUMAN EASE.* The publicity for this compound stated:

"Go Eagle, to All the World and Carry the Glad news of James A. Davis' New Discovery of *HUMAN EASE*. We Guarantee to Cure All Diseases both In and On Man and Beast"

Amongst the diseases cured by *HUMAN EASE* were cancer, syphilis, mad dog bites, ingrowing nails, paralysis, heart disease, smallpox, tuberculosis, obesity and diphtheria. Dr W.S. Hubbard of the Bureau of Chemistry, Department of Agriculture analysed the compound in October 1916, and discovered it to consist of 95.5% lard!!

renowned to be the 'most cruel and conscienceless of the whole crew'. An editorial in a foremost Medical Journal of the time, on Aug 7th 1915 stated "Possibly the human animal can descend to greater depths of depravity than that reached by the cancer quack –

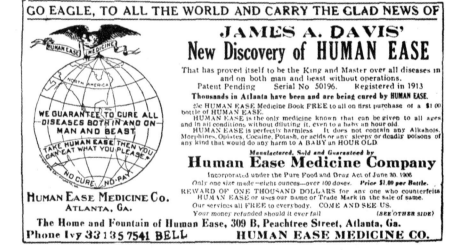

Glossary of terms

3D conformal radiotherapy
External beam radiotherapy that uses a computer generated three-dimensional image of the prostate and special shielding to aim the X ray beam accurately at the cancer

A

Abdomen, abdominal
A part of the body which includes the stomach, intestines and other digestive organs

Abnormal
Not normal – possibly cancerous

Active monitoring
The postponement of treatment whilst regularly monitoring the prostate cancer by measuring the PSA level. Treatment may never be needed. Treatment can have a greater impact on quality of life than prostate cancer itself. The best action can be to monitor the cancer and commence treatment if the situation changes. This can be many years after the first diagnosis. Also called watchful waiting, active surveillance, conservative management, and expectant management

Active surveillance
See Active monitoring

Acupuncture
A complementary therapy and system of healing practised in eastern countries for thousands of years. Fine needles are inserted into 'energy points' just below the skin. Used to treat a wide range of illnesses, it may be given to relieve pain and to treat some side effects of cancer treatments

Adenoma – or polyp
A benign (non-cancerous) tumour having a glandular origin and structure. Can turn cancerous

Adenocarcinoma
A malignant tumour which develops from glandular tissue. The vast majority of prostate cancers are adenocarcinomas. The rest are a variety of much rarer types

Adjuvant therapy
A treatment given as well as the main treatment to help reduce the risk of the cancer returning. Chemotherapy, radiotherapy or hormone therapy can all be used as adjuvant therapies

Advanced prostate cancer
Once prostate cancer has escaped from the prostate gland and spread elsewhere in the body, it is described as advanced. It can be treated using hormone therapy. Also see locally advanced prostate cancer and metastatic cancer

Aggressive
Describes a cancer that is likely to develop and spread quickly

Androgens
Male sex hormones. See testosterone

Anaemia
Any condition in which the blood is deficient in red blood cells or haemoglobin

Anaesthesia, anaesthetics
Drugs or gases given before and during surgery so that the patient will not feel pain. The patient may be awake (local anaesthetic) or asleep (general anaesthetic)

Anti-androgen therapy
A drug treatment that blocks the effects of testosterone, thus stopping it from feeding the prostate cancer. This is a form of hormone therapy

Anti-emetic
A medicine (either tablets, an injection or a drip) that can help you feel less sick

Antioxidant
An antioxidant is a substance that may protect from the damaging effects of free radicals. A diet rich in antioxidants is protective against many forms of cancer and ill health. Antioxidants include zinc and lycopene

Axilla
The armpit

B

Benign
A swelling or growth that is not cancerous, does not spread, and is usually not life-threatening

Bereavement
The period of grief which follows the death of a loved one

Bilateral orchidectomy
An operation where both testicles are removed. See orchidectomy

Biological therapy
Treatment with substances that encourage the body's natural defence system – the immune system – to attack cancer cells. Also known as immunotherapy

Biopsy
One of the main tests used to diagnose cancer. A piece of body tissue is removed from the area where there might be cancer, and the cells are examined under a microscope. This is one of the tests used to decide whether or not a person has cancer, and what type of cancer it is

Bladder
A muscular sac that is connected to the kidneys above. It holds urine which passes out of the bladder and the body through a tube called the urethra

Blood cells
Cells that make up the blood. There are three main types – red blood cells (which carry oxygen around the body), white blood cells (which fight invading germs), and platelets (which help the blood to clot)

Blood count
This shows the number of blood cells in the bloodstream

Bone marrow
The soft and spongy centre of the bone that makes blood cells

Bone scan
A scan which looks for damage to bone

BPH (Benign Prostatic Hyperplasia)
A common condition of the prostate, also know as enlarged prostate. As men get older, the prostate often enlarges. It may grow to a stage where it constricts the urethra causing problems passing urine. It is a separate condition from prostate cancer, but it can exist alongside prostate cancer

Brachytherapy
The insertion of radioactive seeds, or pellets, into a tumour to destroy cancer cells. It is used as treatment for a number of different cancers. The seeds give a dose of radiation directly into the affected area. Brachytherapy is a treatment for localised prostate cancer

Bronchoscopy
A test using a flexible telescope to examine the inside of the lung

C

Cancerous
A term used to describe a tumour which has the ability to spread to nearby organs and tissues, and to other areas of the body

Carcinoma
A type of cancer which begins in the lining or covering of an organ

Catheter
A tube inserted into the bladder through the urethra to assist the flow of urine

Cell
The tiny building blocks which make up all living tissue. Cells can reproduce when needed. They have different structures in different parts of the body

Chemotherapy
Treatment with drugs to kill or slow the growth of cancer cells

Clavicle
The collarbone

Clear margin
An area of normal tissue that surrounds cancerous tissue

Clinician
Hospital doctor

Colectomy
Surgery to remove part of or all of the colon

Colic
A severe spasmodic abdominal pain

Colon
Part of the bowel

Colonoscopy
Visual examination of the inner surface of the colon by means of a flexible tube called a colonoscope

Colorectum, colorectal
Part of the bowel referring to the large intestine

Colostomy
Surgery to attach the colon to the stoma, after the rectum is removed

Complementary therapies
A wide variety of therapies which work alongside conventional medical treatment and focus on improving a person's wellbeing, psychologically as well as physically

Complete androgen blockade (CAB)
A form of hormone therapy where tablets and injections are taken in combination. Another name for MAB

Consultant
Most senior doctor

Conservative management
See active monitoring

Cryotherapy
Also called cryoablation. The use of freezing to destroy cancer cells. This is an uncommon treatment for prostate cancer. A number of probes are inserted into the prostate and liquid nitrogen is used to
freeze and destroy the cancer cells

CT scan
A computed tomography (CT) scan produces a cross-section image of the head and body which is then analysed by a computer

Cystitis
Inflammation of the bladder that causes a burning sensation when peeing

D

Diagnosis
Identifying a disease in a person's body, or deciding what is wrong with them

Digital rectal examination (DRE)
The doctor or nurse feels the prostate gland with a gloved and lubricated finger inserted into the rectum. A DRE helps in the diagnosis of prostate cancer, but is not always diagnostic on its own

E

Endoscopy
Looking inside the body through a small fibre-optic tube

Enlarged prostate
See BPH

Erectile dysfunction
See impotence

Erythrocytes
Red blood cells which carry oxygen from the lungs to cells in all parts of the body and carbon dioxide back from the cells to the lungs

Expectant management
See active monitoring

External beam radiotherapy (EBRT)
A course of high dose X-ray treatment where a beam of radioactive particles is aimed at the cancer from outside the body in order to destroy the cancer

F

Faeces
Poo, number 2, otherwise known as bowel motions. Also see Stool

Fine Needle Aspiration (FNA)
A type of biopsy where a very thin needle is put into a tumour and a sample of fluid and cells is sucked out. The cells are looked at under a microscope to see if they are cancerous

Flare
The body's response to the first hormone therapy injection. The body produces a flush of extra testosterone in response to the injection

Flatus
Wind or a fart

Fraction
A single radiotherapy treatment

Free radicals
A special type of molecule. They can be destructive in the body. Pollution, radiation and other environmental factors can introduce more into the body. Free radicals are believed to be

involved in conditions such as cancer, arthritis, high blood pressure and diabetes. Anti oxidants in the diet may provide some protection against the effects of free radicals

Frequency
The frequent need to pass urine, often just small amounts

G

Genes
The coding material in all cells which affects what they are like and how they behave

Gleason score
Scale that shows how aggressive a prostate cancer is by analysing the type of cells present in a sample. It is important to know this because the score affects the treatment choices. The scale goes from 2- 10, with 2-6 being termed non-aggressive, 7 moderately aggressive and 8-10 aggressive

Guidelines, guidance
Recommended course of action for a particular illness or stage of an illness that is agreed by a team of experts

H

Haemorrhoids
Piles

Hemicolectomy
Removal of half of the colon

Hesitancy
The need to wait a moment or two before the flow of urine starts, even when the bladder is full

Hickman line
A special tube put in under anaesthetic through the chest wall into a large vein, so that chemotherapy drugs can go directly into the bloodstream

High-dose chemotherapy
Using high doses of anti-cancer drugs to kill cancer cells

Hormones
Natural chemicals in the body which affect the way organs and tissues work

Hormone independent
See hormone refractory

Hormone refractory
Sometimes called hormone independent. A state where prostate cancer cells no longer require testosterone to grow and thus grow in its absence. This is when hormone therapy stops being effective

Hormone receptor tests
Laboratory tests which tell if a cancer depends on hormones for growth

Hormone therapy
A treatment that doctors use to try to stop cancer cells from growing by removing, blocking, or adding to the effects of a hormone

Hospice
Specialised units providing palliative care, including symptom control and terminal care, at the final stages of illness

Hot flushes
A common side effect of hormone therapy, similar to the flushes experienced by women going through the menopause. Not all men get them and they vary in severity

I

Ileostomy
Removal of colon and rectum, attachment of the bottom of the small intestine to the stoma

Immune system
The body's natural defence system against infection or disease

Immunotherapy
Treatment with substances that encourage the body's natural defence system – the immune system – to attack cancer cells. Also known as biological therapy

Implant
Something put into the body for a period of time, sometimes permanently

Inoperable
Refers to a cancer that cannot be removed by surgery

Impotence
Inability to achieve an erection firm enough for sexual intercourse to take place. This is sometimes referred to as ED or erectile dysfunction

Incontinence
Involuntary loss of urine at inconvenient moments. This may be slight, when a pad has to be used to protect against a few drops that leak out occasionally. It may be more severe and require a catheter – a tube passed into the bladder –and attached to a leg bag, to make sure the urine drains safely and discreetly

Infusion
Introduction of fluid or medicines (such as chemotherapy drugs) into an artery or vein

In situ
The earliest stage of cancer, when it has not spread to any other organ or area of the body

Intra-muscular
Injection into a muscle

Intravenous (IV)
Injection into a vein

Invasive
A cancer which spreads to nearby tissue

L

Latent period
Interval between the beginning of a disease and the time that the patients gets symptoms or realises there is something wrong. There can be a long latent period in prostate cancer

Laxative
Over-the-counter medicine to soften constipated stools

Lead-time bias
If someone is screened for a disease, and the disease is found sooner than it would have been if you waited for symptoms to appear, the amount of time by which diagnosis moves forwards is the lead-time. As the point of diagnosis is then advanced in time, survival, as measured from diagnosis, is automatically lengthened, even if total length of life is not

Leukaemia
Cancer of the white blood cells

Leukocytes
White blood cells that defend the body against infections and other diseases

Lobe, lobule
Part of an organ or gland in the body

LHRH agonist
(Luteinizing Hormone-Releasing Hormone) hormone therapy drug used in advanced prostate cancer, usually injected into the abdomen, which causes a reduction in testosterone production and thus shrinks the cancer. LHRH agonists include Zoladex, Prostap, Suprefact and De-Capeptyl

Libido
Sex drive or desire. May be severely affected by hormone therapy

Lump
A lump that can be felt under the skin may be a sign of cancer, but most are not cancerous

Localised prostate cancer
Prostate cancer that remains entirely within the gland and has the best chance of being cured

Locally advanced prostate cancer
A locally advanced cancer is one that is no longer confined entirely to the prostate, but has not gone far. It is not found in bone, or in local lymph nodes

Lumpectomy
Surgically removing a lump and a small amount of tissue around it

Lycopene
A powerful antioxidant found in tomatoes, which may reduce the chance of prostate cancer developing. Processed tomatoes, especially in tomato sauce, are especially rich in it. It is also found in other red fruits and vegetables, for example strawberries

Lymphatic system
The system that removes waste from body tissues, filters lymphatic fluid and produces cells that fight infection

Lymph nodes
Small bean-shaped organs, sometimes called lymph glands, which are part of the lymphatic system

Lymphocyte
A type of white blood cell which protects against infection

Lymphoedema
Swelling in the arms or legs that is caused when the lymph vessels are blocked or damaged. This can be caused by treatments for cancer or by the cancer itself

Lymphoma
A cancer of the lymph glands or lymphatic system

M

Malignant
Capable of invading, spreading and destroying tissue

Maximal androgen blockade (MAB)
Form of hormone therapy where tablets and injections are taken in combination. Another name for CAB

Medical oncologist
Medical doctor specialising in the treatment of cancer

Meditation
A method of relaxation

Metastasis, metastasise, metastatic
The spread of cancer cells from one part of the body to another through the bloodstream or lymphatic system. Cells that have metastasised are like those in the original tumour

Micro-calcifications
Tiny deposits of calcium that may show that cancer is present

Monitoring
Regularly checking up to see how a patient is doing or responding to treatment

MRI scan
A magnetic resonance imaging (MRI) scan uses magnets to produce pictures, which are then analysed by a computer

N

Nausea
Feeling sick

Neoplasm
Another word for cancer. From the Latin for "new growth" neoplasia – neo = new; plasia = growth

Nocturia
The need to get up to urinate during the night

Node
Part of the lymphatic system, which is the body's natural defence against infection. Lymph nodes are small masses of tissue found in clusters which purify the lymph fluid and form lymphocytes (white blood cells)

Nutrition
A healthy diet and the correct intake of vitamins and minerals. This can be difficult to achieve for some people with cancer and they may need advice from health professionals

O

Oedema
A build-up of fluid in part of the body

Oesophagus, oesophageal
A tube from the mouth to the stomach

Oestrogen
Female sex hormone. This may be used in hormone therapy to reduce the body's production of testosterone

Oncology
The study and treatment of cancer

Orally
Given by mouth

Orchidectomy
Removal of the testicles, popularly known as castration. A treatment for advanced prostate cancer. The operation stops the production of most testosterone, the male hormone that feeds the cancer

Ostomist
A person who has a stoma

Osteoporosis
Bone thinning due to age, level of exercise or through hormonal change. This may be associated with taking hormone therapy to treat advanced prostate cancer

P

Palliative care
Palliative care is designed to relieve symptoms rather than cure. It can be used at any stage of the illness if there are symptoms such as pain or sickness. Palliative care may help someone to live longer and to live comfortably, even if they cannot be cured

Pancreas
An organ in the digestive system that makes insulin and some of the enzymes needed for digesting food

Pathology
Examining tissues, particularly the changes in cells and tissues resulting from disease

Polyp
Mass of tissue that bulges or projects outward or upward from the surface of the bowel lining

Peripheral blood stem cell transplant (PBSCT)
A procedure in which stem cells are removed from the patient's blood, stored and then put back into the bloodstream

Perineum
The area of the body between the back of the scrotum and the anus

Platelets
The blood cells which prevent bleeding by causing blood to clot at the site of an injury

Primary cancer
Where the cancer first started in the body

Primary care
Usually used to refer to health services provided in the community rather than in hospital (for example, general practice or district nursing)

Proctitis
Inflammation of the rectum

Prognosis
The predicted or likely outcome of what might happen in a specific case of cancer

Prostate, prostatic
A gland found only in men, under the bladder. It produces fluid which forms part of semen and helps nourish sperm

Prostatitis
A range of problems in the prostate gland, related to inflammation and infection

Prostatectomy
Surgical removal of the whole, or part of the prostate. A radical prostatectomy is removal of the entire prostate gland and is a treatment for prostate cancer. Operations for BPH, or for severe urinary symptoms due to prostate cancer, may remove only part of the gland. See TURP

Prognosis
Expected outcome or end result of treatment. Often used to mean life expectancy

Prosthesis
An artificial replacement of part of the body

PSA (prostate specific antigen)
A special kind of protein called an enzyme, produced by the prostate gland. It is normal to find some in the blood stream of men

PSA test
Blood test to check the levels of PSA. It helps in diagnosis, and also in monitoring the effects of treatment

R

Radiation therapy, radiotherapy
A treatment which uses high-energy x-rays to kill cancer cells or keep them from dividing and growing

Radical prostatectomy
Operation to remove the entire prostate gland to treat prostate cancer – see prostatectomy

Receptor test
A laboratory test used to work out if a cancer depends on a certain hormone for growth

Recurrence
The return of cancer cells and signs of cancer after they appear to have gone. Sometimes known as a relapse

Reflexology
A complementary therapy which can be used as well as medical cancer treatment. It involves massaging areas of the feet

Regression
When a cancer has shrunk or disappeared

Remission
A person is said to be 'in remission' when their cancer stops growing or shows no symptoms

Rectum
The final part of the digestive system before the anus

Risk factor
An aspect of personal behaviour or lifestyle, or an environmental exposure or inherited characteristic known to be associated with a health problem e.g. smoking is a risk factor because it increases your risk of heart disease. A high fat diet seems to be risk factor for prostate cancer

S

Screening
The routine examination of apparently health people, to identify those with a particular disease at an early stage, before anyone could be aware of it through symptoms

Secondaries, secondary cancer
New tumours, or metastases, which are formed because cancer cells from the original tumour have been carried to other parts of the body

Seminal vesicles
The two sacs at the base of the bladder in men that produce seminal fluid. They are connected to the prostate gland

Sentinel lymph node
The first lymph nodes that cancer cells spread to after leaving the area of the primary tumour

Shiatsu
A type of gentle massage which works on the energy flow around the body and can be helpful for stress-related conditions

Sigmoid
Last bit of the colon, above the rectum

Stage
A classification of a cancer according to its size and how much it has spread

Staging
Working out how much the cancer has spread. It is helpful when deciding on the best treatment options

Stem cell
The immature cells in blood and bone marrow from which all mature blood cells develop

Stoma
An artificial opening between an organ and the skin surface, that is formed by surgery. For example, a colostomy is an opening to the colon

Stool
Discharge of the bowels, the digestive waste matter discharged at one movement of the bowels; also called faeces

Sub-capsular orchidectomy
Operation where the part of the testicle that produces testosterone is removed. This leaves the outside shell of the testicle in place, preserving the external appearance. See orchidectomy

Subcutaneous
Given by injection under the skin

Surgery
An operation

Syringe drivers
A way of giving painkilling or chemotherapy drugs under the skin which means that patients do not need to have regular injections

Systemic therapy
Using treatments, such as chemotherapy, that affect the whole body

T

Terminal care
Caring for a person in the last days or weeks before they die, making sure they are free of pain and as comfortable as possible

Testosterone
Male sex hormone, or androgen. Amongst other functions, testosterone controls the growth, development and regeneration of cells in the prostate gland

Therapy
Treatment

Thoracic
Referring to the chest area

Tissue
A group of cells

Tumour
A group of abnormal cells which keep on growing, crowding out normal cells

Tumour markers
Substances produced by some cancers that can be traced in the blood

TURP (Trans Urethral Resection of the Prostate):
Surgical procedure where the inside of the prostate is removed through the urethra. This is an operation to relieve symptoms such as difficulty passing urine. Used in the treatment of BPH and sometimes to relive urinary symptoms in prostate cancer

U

Ultrasound scan
A scan which uses sound waves to build up an image of the internal organs

Urethra
The tube that carries urine from the bladder and semen from the reproductive system through the penis to the outside of the body

Urgency
The strong need to urinate, almost immediately

Urology
Surgical speciality dealing with th urinary tract – in men this is the kidneys, bladder, prostate, penis and testicles

W

Watchful waiting
See active monitoring

X

X-ray
A high-energy form of radiation. It is used in low doses to diagnose diseases and in high doses to treat cancer
back to top

Y

Yoga
A combination of relaxation, breathing techniques and exercise to help deal with stress and improve circulation and movement of the joints

Index

Editor	Ian Barnes
Editorial director	Matthew Minter
Front cover picture	Mark Stevens
Page build	James Robertson
Production control	Kevin Heals
Technical illustrations	Roger Healing and Mark Stevens

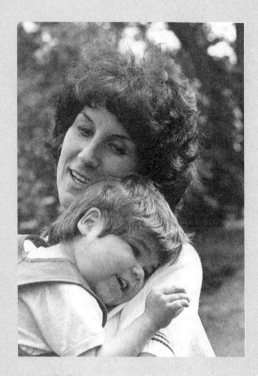

The Anthony Nolan Trust exists to *"facilitate a transplant for any patient in the world in need of bone marrow or appropriate cells"*.

The Anthony Nolan Trust (ANT) maintains the UK's largest register of over 330,000 potential volunteer donors willing to donate their blood stem cells should their tissue type match that of a patient in need of transplant to help fight leukaemia or other immune deficiency diseases.

In addition ANT research programmes constantly work to improve the outcome of bone marrow transplantation and have also made a major contribution to advances in the field of leukaemia research and treatment.

We need public support in two vital areas: -

<u>Joining the Anthony Nolan Trust Register</u> – the more people that are on the register and willing to donate if a suitable match is found, the better the chances of a successful transplant for one of thousands of patients around the world currently waiting for treatment.

If you are aged between 18 and 40, in good general health and willing to become a volunteer donor, please contact the Trust. We urge all eligible volunteers to come forward, but have a specific clinical need to recruit more male, ethnic minority and mixed race volunteers. To find out more please call the ANT on 020 7284 1234.

<u>Fundraising</u> – ANT receives no Government funding and is totally reliant on voluntary support to maintain its donor register and research work. If you would like to invest in our vital work there are several ways to make a donation; you can find out more by visiting our web site at <u>www.anthonynolan.org.uk</u>.

You can also show your support by participating in local fundraising events. Whether you're in the north, south, east or west of the UK, we have the event for you! You can choose to take part in an overwhelming variety of events, from a sponsored walk in your local park to a more adventurous trek in a remote or exotic location. To find out more visit our web site at <u>www.anthonynolan.org.uk</u> and follow the links to the fundraising pages.

Whatever way you decide to help, we value your contribution to our charity.
Thank you for your support.

THE ANTHONY NOLAN TRUST

Where leukaemia meets its match

Any question on any cancer, in your language

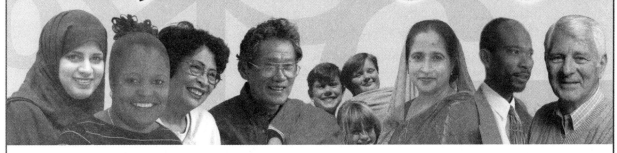

Our confidential freephone language helplines offer support and information to anyone affected by cancer.

للحصول على معلومات عن مرض السرطان بالعربية يرجى الاتصال ب
0808 800 0130 (Arabic)

বাংলায় ক্যান্সার বিষয়ে তথ্যের জন্য ফোন করুন:
0808 800 0131 (Bengali)

有關癌症的資訊（粵語），請致電：
0808 800 0132 (Cantonese)

Pour toute information en français sur le cancer veuillez appeler le :
0808 800 0133 (French)

Για πληροφορίες στην ελληνική γλώσσα για θέματα που αφορούν τον καρκίνο καλέστε:
0808 800 0134 (Greek)

કેન્સર બાબત ગુજરાતીમાં માહિતી મેળવવા માટે, ટેલિફોન કરો:
0808 800 0135 (Gujarati)

केन्सर के बारे में हिन्दी में जानकारी पाने के लिये, टैलिफ़ोन करें :
0808 800 0136 (Hindi)

W języku polskim informację o chorobach raka uzyskasz telefonicznie pod Nr:
0808 800 0137 (Polish)

ਕੈਂਸਰ ਦੇ ਬਾਰੇ ਪੰਜਾਬੀ 'ਚ ਜਾਣਕਾਰੀ ਪ੍ਰਾਪਤ ਕਰਨ ਲਈ, ਟੈਲਿਫ਼ੋਨ ਕਰੋ:
0808 800 0138 (Punjabi)

Kanserle ilgili Türkçe bilgi için,
0808 800 0139 (Turkish)

اردو میں کینسر کے متعلق معلومات کے لئے فون کریں:
0808 800 0140 (Urdu)

Để có được các thông tin về bệnh ung thư bằng tiếng Việt, xin quí vị gọi số:
0808 800 0141 (Vietnamese)

For cancer information in any language call freephone: **0808 800 1234**

New Opportunities Fund
LOTTERY FUNDED

www.cancerbacup.org.uk

cancerBACUP
helping people live with cancer

Charity No: 1019719

TRUST ME, I'M A ~~DOCTOR~~
CANCER PATIENT

'You will cope better because you know what to expect' someone once said to me. I did not know what to expect, I had never been a cancer patient before.

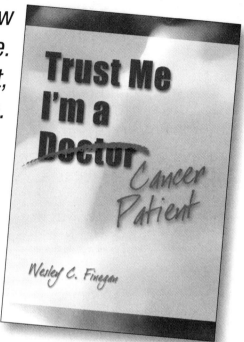

Dr Wesley C Finegan was diagnosed with cancer ten years ago whilst working as a consultant in palliative medicine, giving him a unique perspective as a cancer patient. In this enlightening work, he offers practical and sensible advice, encouraging patients to work with doctors and nurses to deal with common issues, including pain, and the physical, personal, social and spiritual problems which can occur when suffering from cancer.

Typical problems include:

- What do I need to know about my pain?
- I've lost my appetite
- I am breathless
- I have a dry mouth
- I am having nightmares
- I am feeling sick
- I am having difficulty swallowing
- I am feeling weak
- How do I tell my children the bad news?
- How do I tell others the bad news?
- I would like to try complementary (alternative) therapy
- I want to make a will
- I would like to return to work
- I want to think about my spiritual needs

The book can be read from cover to cover, or can be dipped into for quick reference whenever needed.

2004 192 pages Paper, £14.95 ISBN 1 85775 877 3

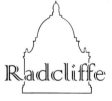

malehealth

a unique health website

fast, free independent info from the Men's Health Forum

Want to find out more?

malehealth.co.uk is a new health website aimed at blokes of all ages - it aims to bring you the information you want in a form that's easy to read and even easier to find.

At its heart is a Key Info section which covers 24 common health topics in a clear Q and A format. It includes, for beginners, the Male Body - A User's Guide, an overview of every part of the male anatomy.

You can get an instant online health report and we'll talk you through how to do a home MOT health check. Then there's frank healthy living advice in the Easy Ways to Feel Better section including all our favourite subjects: drink, smoking, sex, food and exercise. And, for those who want a more detailed work-out, there is our online gym including a seven week fitness programme specially designed by Britain's most capped athlete. On top of all that, there's news, features, statistics and links to useful books and other web-sites.

Register for a free newsletter to get all the latest updates. It all adds up to a very comprehensive site - so far as we know, the only one of its type in the world.

The site is run by the Men's Health Forum, the leading voluntary organisation working to improve men's health in the UK, of which Dr Ian Banks is president. So take Dr Ian's advice: prescribe yourself a visit to malehealth today.

Look forward to seeing you,

Jim Pollard, editor, malehealth.co.uk

www.malehealth.co.uk

Preserving Our Motoring Heritage

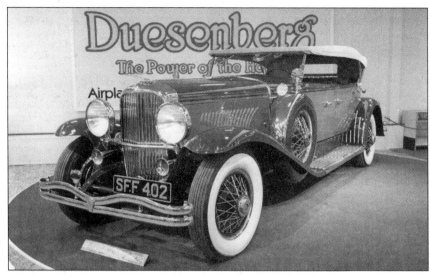

< *The Model J Duesenberg Derham Tourster. Only eight of these magnificent cars were ever built – this is the only example to be found outside the United States of America*

Almost every car you've ever loved, loathed or desired is gathered under one roof at the Haynes Motor Museum. Over 300 immaculately presented cars and motorbikes represent every aspect of our motoring heritage, from elegant reminders of bygone days, such as the superb Model J Duesenberg to curiosities like the bug-eyed BMW Isetta. There are also many old friends and flames. Perhaps you remember the 1959 Ford Popular that you did your courting in? The magnificent 'Red Collection' is a spectacle of classic sports cars including AC, Alfa Romeo, Austin Healey, Ferrari, Lamborghini, Maserati, MG, Riley, Porsche and Triumph.

A Perfect Day Out

Each and every vehicle at the Haynes Motor Museum has played its part in the history and culture of Motoring. Today, they make a wonderful spectacle and a great day out for all the family. Bring the kids, bring Mum and Dad, but above all bring your camera to capture those golden memories for ever. You will also find an impressive array of motoring memorabilia, a comfortable 70 seat video cinema and one of the most extensive transport book shops in Britain. The Pit Stop Cafe serves everything from a cup of tea to wholesome, home-made meals or, if you prefer, you can enjoy the large picnic area nestled in the beautiful rural surroundings of Somerset.

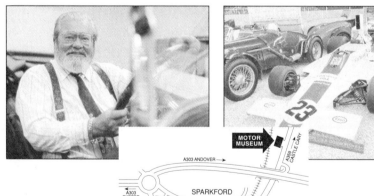

John Haynes O.B.E., Founder and Chairman of the museum at the wheel of a Haynes Light 12. >

< *Graham Hill's Lola Cosworth Formula 1 car next to a 1934 Riley Sports.*

The Museum is situated on the A359 Yeovil to Frome road at Sparkford, just off the A303 in Somerset. It is about 40 miles south of Bristol, and 25 minutes drive from the M5 intersection at Taunton.
Open 9.30am - 5.30pm (10.00am - 4.00pm Winter) 7 days a week, *except Christmas Day, Boxing Day and New Years Day*
Special rates available for schools, coach parties and outings Charitable Trust No. 292048